The Whole Foods Plant Based Cookbook for Longevity

Plant Based Healthy Meal Prep Featuring a 10 Day Eat Real Food Plan

Paul Griggs

Your FREE Book Bonus!

As a show of appreciation for reading this book here is a link to your free book bonus, *The Whole Foods Plant Based Recipes Kickstarter*:

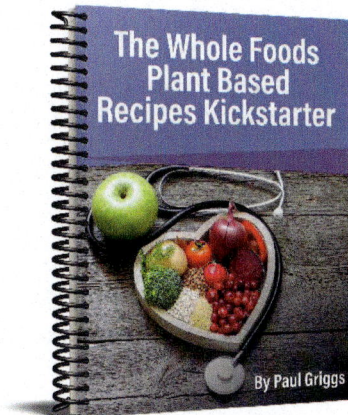

https://paulgriggs.aweb.page/kickstarter

Inside you will find more delicious recipes for appetizers, brunch, and dinner, to enhance your 10 day eat real food plan!

"Eat food. Not too much. Mostly plants."

- Michael Pollan
Harvard Professor, bestselling author of *Omnivore's Dilemma*, speaker on food and health

"[People living past 100] don't eat high quantity meat or cheese. They don't eat heaps of sugar. They consume lots of complex carbs like beans and vegetables with plenty of healthy fats from olive oil and nuts."

- Dr. Valter Longo
Director of The Longevity Institute

"For the vast majority of chronic diseases, it's the same lifestyle recommendations... essentially a whole foods, plant-based diet."

-   Dr. Dean Ornish
President of the Preventive Medicine Research Institute, bestselling author of *The Spectrum* and *Undo It*

Contents

Introduction 1

Tips to ease your transition to plant-based 2

Sugar, Oil, and Salt (SOS) 3

Chapter 1 8

Tips for Transitioning to a Plant-Based Kitchen 8

Whole foods plant-based weekly shopping list 8

Plant-based kitchen tools 11

Chapter 2 13

Sample Meals 13

Breakfast is optional! 13

Breakfast of Tofu Champions 13

Spinach Omelet 15

Gingerbread Waffles 17

Smoothies 19

Peanut dream smoothie 19

Chocolate Peanut Butter Banana Smoothie 20

Super Green Smoothie 22

Blueberry Smoothie Bowl 24

Salads and Bowls 26

Arugula Quinoa Bowl 26

Quinoa Salad 28

Ancient Grains Bowl (from True Food Kitchen) 30

Quinoa Gado-Gado Bowl 32

Black Bean and Avocado Bowl 34

Tempeh Salad with Brussels Sprouts 36

Chickpea and Sweet Potato Salad 38

Corn and Black Bean Salad 40

Pastas.. 41

Savory sausage pasta 41

Vegan Lasagna 43

Vegan Spicy Sausage Pasta......................................45

Spaghetti with Beyond Meatballs 47

Creamy mushroom risotto 49

Polish Inspired 51

Vegan haluski - polish comfort food 51

American Inspired.. 53

Chef special! Mom's herb-crusted meatloaf.............53

Mexican Inspired 55

Mexican bean salad 55

Vegan Enchilada Skillet.. 57

Bean and Tomato Casserole 59

Black Bean Burritos 62

Caribbean Inspired..64

Cuban Black Bean Soup.. 64

Asian Inspired 66

"Chicken" Teriyaki 66

Pad Thai with tofu..68

Chow Mein - Vegan...71

Curry Cauliflower Soup... 73

Sweet Potato, Spinach, and Lentil Dhal...................75

American Favorites 77

Award winning! Ultimate vegan chili 77

Black Bean Burgers...80

Live Long and Strong pizza.....................................80

Desserts - yes you can make desserts without dairy! 82

Banana Energy Cookies 82

Dairy-Free Pineapple Whip......................................84

Peanut butter cookies..*86*

Chapter 3..**88**
Ten Days to Transform Your Health: The 10 Day Eat Real Food Plan **88**

Breakfast..90

Lunch recipes 91

Day 1: Mexican bean salad.............................. 91

Day 2: Black Bean Burritos.............................. 92

Day 3: Garden Salad 93

Day 4: "Chicken" Teriyaki 93

Day 5: Ancient Grains Bowl (from True Food Kitchen) 96

Day 6: Black Bean and Avocado Bowl.............. 97

Day 7: Quinoa Gado-Gado Bowl....................98

Day 8: Arugula Quinoa Bowl.......................... 99

Day 9: Pad Thai with tofu 100

Day 10: Chow Mein.. 102

Dinner Recipes 103

Day 1: Savory sausage pasta 103

Day 2: Chef special! Mom's herb-crusted meatloaf.. 104

Day 3: Vegan haluski - polish comfort food 105

Day 4: Award winning! Ultimate vegan chili 106

Day 5: Spaghetti with Beyond Meatballs 108

Day 6: Black Bean Burgers 109

Day 7: Brown Rice Stir Fry 110

Day 8: Garden Pizza....................................... 111

Day 9: Creamy mushroom risotto 113

Day 10: Cuban Black Bean Soup....................114

Conclusion **116**

Introduction

Welcome to Book 2 in this series! You may have decided to eat plant-based for your health and lifespan, to enjoy more time with those you love. Science shows eating plant-based lowers your risk of cardiovascular disease and cancer, the leading causes of premature death. Cardiovascular diseases include high blood pressure, diabetes, high cholesterol, and heart disease, all of which increase risk of heart attacks. If someone you love is not well, they might also make diet changes to reverse cardiovascular diseases and reduce medication costs and side effects. Readers interested in scientific research supporting whole foods, plant-based eating are referred to *The Whole Foods Diet for Longevity*.

You may also choose a plant-based diet for peak performance, or environmental reasons like optimizing water, land, and energy use and reducing global warming. Or you may want to eat plant-based to reduce animal cruelty. Whatever your reason, welcome to a growing share of the population leading a plant-based lifestyle!

Before you start any healthy meal prep in the pages that follow, a few friendly reminders from *The Whole Foods Diet for Longevity*. First, a whole foods plant-based diet does not include meat, dairy, and seafood. This is recommended by some of the highest authorities on diet: Dr. Dean Ornish, Dr. Neal Barnard, Harvard Nutrition studies, etc. However, this doesn't mean you limit yourself to lettuce and tomatoes. You can eat an abundance of whole plant foods: fruits, vegetables, whole grains, legumes, and some nuts and seeds.

Second, you aren't going to need a calculator because there is no need to count carbs or calories! A lot of people LOVE this one! For example, you could eat plenty of fruit salad and peanut butter granola. Eating bland foods is not required. Experiment with all the spices and seasonings you like!

Most people stop using the "diet" label and begin using "lifestyle." Maybe this is because of the notion that "diets" are too confusing and warped. It brings up images of struggling and framing every meal as one more challenge to win against. A whole foods plant-based (vegan) lifestyle is completely different. It is not a short-term punishment that makes you feel guilty. It is simply turning back to natural health, rich flavor, and whole foods.

Tips to ease your transition to plant-based

Keep in mind these recommended daily serving sizes of the six health-promoting whole foods, from Harvard Nutrition and the Alternate Healthy Eating Index (see Book 1 Chapter 3).

Health-promoting food	Daily serving size
Water	2.5-3.5L for mild to moderate activity, more when hot
Fruit	4 servings (4 cups) antioxidant-rich, may include berries for fiber
Vegetables	5 servings (400g) antioxidant-rich, 1 serving cruciferous: broccoli sprouts, brussels sprouts, cabbage, cauliflower, kale, etc.
Whole grains	6 servings (3 cups cooked), should be the largest part of your plate for fiber
Nuts/seeds	1 serving (30g), top source of omega 3s, plant protein, remember nut milk, nut butter

Legumes	4-5 servings (2 cups) for fiber and plant protein

Notice daily food recommendations do not include foods lowest in antioxidants: seafood, meat, dairy, and eggs.[1] This is also recommended by Dr. Ornish, who recommends eating only plant protein based on 40 years of nutrition research.[2] He concluded that chronic diseases like heart disease, diabetes, and cancer are caused by oxidative stress and inflammation (see Book 1 Chapter 2). This means **you want to eat an abundance of antioxidant foods. The top antioxidant foods are listed in the table.**

Of course, how quickly you transition to a whole foods plant-based diet is your choice. I cut dairy first, got good results, then cut meat. Many people start out by cutting meat first, keeping dairy and fish, then slowly transition to whole foods plant-based.

Sugar, Oil, and Salt (SOS)

Many people have heard it's healthy to reduce sugar, oil, and salt consumption. That is a half-truth. Dr. Ornish says the healthiest diet is "a whole foods, plant-based diet naturally low in refined carbs." He recommends "replacing refined carbs (processed foods) with healthy carbs like fruits, vegetables, whole grains and legumes for anti-heart disease,

---

[1] See Chapter 3 in *The Whole Foods Diet for Longevity* and Table 1 in Carlsen, M et al. (2010). The total antioxidant content of more than 3100 foods, beverages, spices, herbs and supplements used worldwide. *Nutrition Journal*, 9(1). https://doi.org/10.1186/1475-2891-9-3

[2] For more on protein, see Chapter 1 in *The Whole Foods Diet for Longevity*

anti-cancer, and anti-aging properties."[3] In other words, you would want to replace refined sugars like white pasta, white rice, pizza, baked goods with white or brown sugar, etc. with whole foods for a healthy, long life. Remember, carbs do not cause you to gain fat; eating refined carbs causes you to gain fat and is associated with obesity.[4]

So you do not want to eat a low carb diet. For healthy weight and long life you want to eat zero *refined* carbs. The health-promoting whole foods have healthy sugar that fuels all the cells in your body (complex carbs). This is why **people living over 100 eat a high carbohydrate diet**, per Dr. Longo.

How healthy is oil? When cooking stir fry vegetables, or caramelizing onions and garlic, remember to **avoid trans fats from hydrogenated vegetable oils**. If you buy cooking oils that are "partially hydrogenated" you are buying toxic, saturated trans fats. Per Harvard nutrition, you should replace saturated fats (like beef and dairy fat) with unsaturated fats.[5] You may remember one of the top sources of essential omega 3 fat (ALA) is canola oil. [6]   Instead of unhealthy hydrogenated oil, **you could choose cold-pressed canola oil for unsaturated fats rich in omega 3s.** You may remember Dr. Longo, Director of the Longevity Institute, a leader in research on age-related

---

3 Robbins, Tony et al. (2022). *Life Force: How New Breakthroughs in Precision Medicine Can Transform the Quality of Your Life & Those You Love.* Simon & Schuster. pg 280-281

4 Spadaro, P, et al (2015). A refined high carbohydrate diet is associated with changes in the serotonin pathway and visceral obesity. *Genetics Research*, 97. https://doi.org/10.1017/s0016672315000233

5 *Types of Fat*. (2018, July 24). The Nutrition Source. https://www.hsph.harvard.edu/nutritionsource/what-should-you-eat-fats-and-cholesterol/types-of-fat/

6 see *The Whole Foods Diet for Longevity*, Chapter 3

disease. Per Dr. Longo's research on living over 100, if you want to live a long life, you could use cold-pressed olive oil. [7] Cold-pressed canola oil and olive oil are healthy fats.

What about salt? The highest sources of salt for Americans are chicken, cheese, and white bread. Eating these sodium-rich foods is the main contributing factor to double the daily recommended intake, per the American Heart Association. [8]

A 2011 study showed people with a higher ratio of sodium to potassium had twice the risk of death by heart attack and a 50% higher risk of death overall. [9]   In this study, people with the highest potassium intake showed a 20% lower risk of death. **This means you want to avoid sodium-rich foods like chicken, cheese, and white bread, replacing them with potassium-rich whole foods like fruits and vegetables.**

Should you use table salt or sea salt? Table salt has low mineral value as it's just sodium and chloride. Iodized salt adds the mineral iodine. Per Harvard nutrition, sea salt has more essential minerals that interact with other nutrients for optimal health and peak performance, including potassium, iron, and zinc. [10]   Since sea salt gives you more essential minerals you want, it is healthy to include sea salt as part of

---

[7] *See The Whole Foods Diet for Longevity* Chapters 1-2

[8] *Jessica Caporusio, Pharm D. (2019, October 2). What is the difference between sea salt and table salt?* https://www.medicalnewstoday.com/articles/326519#intake-recommendations

[9] Yang, Q et al. (2011). Sodium and potassium intake and mortality among US adults. *Archives of Internal Medicine, 171*(13), 1183. https://doi.org/10.1001/archinternmed.2011.257

[10] *Salt and sodium.* (2023, June 13). The Nutrition Source. https://www.hsph.harvard.edu/nutritionsource/salt-and-sodium/

your seasoning. Like fruits and vegetables, it is a potassium source that lowers your risk of heart attack death.

It's true you want to avoid certain types of sugar, oil, and salt. The whole truth is there are healthy alternatives for refined carbs, saturated fat, and high salt foods like chicken and cheese. You can replace refined carbs like white bread with whole grain bread. You can replace hydrogenated cooking oil with healthy fats like canola or olive oil. You can replace high salt chicken and cheese with potassium-rich whole foods including fruits and vegetables. You can also replace table salt with sea salt for seasoning.

Remember, for healthy carbs you want whole grains. The easiest way to find whole grains is to look for "whole" as the first word in the nutrition label: whole grain pasta, whole grain bread, whole wheat crackers, etc. You could also use brown rice, quinoa, and corn on the cob. If you want tastier than brown rice, you can use legumes, e.g. lentils.

Time-saving tips for busy cooks

As you add legumes to your diet, you can start with canned beans and lentils as these do not need to be soaked overnight before eating. Lentils do not require any soaking time, just rinse, then simmer for 15 minutes and add sea salt to taste. It's faster and tastier than brown rice! If you make a whole 1lb package, you can store half in the fridge for a few days and simply combine with cooked grains later to save time. Every time you add legumes to grains, it enriches the texture and flavor of the grain. You might consider adding lentils to your rice, quinoa, or corn. Everyone has heard of rice and beans. This is healthier, tastier brown rice and lentils.

So let's get cooking! In Chapter 1 we will review more tips to stock your kitchen with some of the most common foods you'll need for healthy meal prep. This will be done using a time-tested plant-based shopping list used to make my favorite recipes in this book. We will also recommend plant-based cooking tools.

In Chapter 2 you will discover 28 kitchen-tested savory recipes. You will find many meals look more like Asian food, but you can also use plant-based ground to make Italian, American, and other foods (Beyond Meat and Impossible brands). Remember fourteen of the NFL Titans defense players continued eating delicious meals using plant-based chicken and cheese substitutes (see Book 1 Chapter 5).

For lunch you could have juicy black bean burritos. Or you could have bowlfuls of delicious Pad Thai or mouth-watering Mexican Bean Salad. Would you like gourmet cuisine? Try the Bean and Tomato Casserole bursting with flavor from cherry tomatoes and shallots, mixed between layers of crunchy toasted bread, topped with a cashew parmesan and caper gremolata!

For dinner you might have vegan garlic toast followed by Savory Sausage Pasta. You could have Herb-Crusted Meatloaf or Creamy Mushroom Risotto. Or, you can have award-winning Ultimate Chili…

In Chapter 3 you will discover your Ten Day Eat Real Food Plan. Remember, there is a ten day meal guide here, but you don't have to limit yourself to just ten days. The goal here is to give you ten days of savory plant-based meals from around the world. The link to bonus content at the beginning of this book will give you more recipes. Be on the lookout for an upcoming book in this series with many, many more!

Chapter 1

Tips for Transitioning to a Plant-Based Kitchen

"It's essentially a whole foods, plant-based diet naturally low in fat and refined carbs."

- Dr. Dean Ornish, President of the Preventive Medicine Research Institute, in Life Force

What does it take to prepare plant-based meals? If you want to prepare plant-based meals, you need a plant-based kitchen. Here's a time-tested plant-based shopping list to ensure you have everything you need for healthy meal prep each week. This list of whole foods feeds a 220lb athlete, so you can scale down based on your weight and activity level. Readers interested in weekly or monthly pricing are referred to Chapter 6 in *The Whole Foods Diet for Longevity*.

Whole foods plant-based weekly shopping list

Table 1: Weekly shopping list for a 220lb male athlete

Meals	Whole Foods items you need for Healthy Meal Prep
breakfast	JustEgg replacer
	juice (berry or pineapple) 1.89L
	granola with whole oats, e.g. Bear Naked Peanut Butter

	almond milk with vanilla 2L
	6 bananas
	whole grain loaf / raisin bread loaf
lunch	Chipotle bean burrito no dairy
dinner	bread baguette for vegan garlic toast
	canola or olive oil 1L
	vidalia or spanish onion (2), garlic
	spices: basil, sage, garlic salt, sea salt, pepper
	2lb frozen veggies, 2lb frozen corn
	kale / spinach power greens for salad
	Italian salad dressing
	1lb brussels sprouts / stir fry veggies
	brown rice precooked 1 box
	chili beans, 3 cans (for Ultimate Chili twice a month)
	celery or peppers
	Beyond Meat plant-based ground 1lb (serves 3)
	marinara sauce 1 jar lasts 2mo
	red lentils 1lb
	plant ground Impossible sausage 1lb
	whole grain pasta 2lb

	rice noodles 1lb for vegan haluski
	vegan butter, e.g. Earth Balance
	vegetable gyoza
	Food when you don't have time to cook
	potatoes, two 1lb bags (roasted with peppers and onions Trader Joe's)
	mixed nuts 1lb (walnuts, pecans, almonds)
	graham crackers 1lb box
	Natural peanut butter 1kg lasts two months
	corn chips 1lb
	medium salsa 1 jar
	lemonade 1 gal
	grapes 2lb
	strawberries 1lb
	mixed fruit cans (3.5 servings/can pineapple, pear, cherry)
	tangerines 3lb bag
	cantaloupe, whole
	peanuts, roasted 2lb

* eating whole foods plant-based, 2400 calories in two meals and snacks each day, fruit only before noon

You may want to take this list with you for groceries a few times while you're transitioning to a plant-based lifestyle. You can see the emphasis on whole foods: fruit, vegetables, whole grains, and legumes. For anyone with diabetes, this is the plant-based diet shown to lower blood sugar three times more than a meat-based diet (see Chapter 2 in Book 1).

Please note this shopping list provides 2400 calories per day for an adult male athlete, as opposed to the 2000 calories per day recommended for women. If you weigh under 220lb or are female, this list may sustain you for two full weeks. It may feed a child for up to a month.

Plant-based kitchen tools

You may also want to invest in some cooking tools. For example, if you like smoothies, or you like pasta and want to make your own vegan cheeses, you would want a high quality blender. This would be at a higher price point than your typical $40 blender, e.g. Oster base model. I love smoothies and could eat cashew cheese by itself! To this end, my preferred blender is a Vitamix blender. If you want to make pizzas you would also need a high end blender to make the pesto sauce for Live Long and Strong Pizza (otherwise you will find yourself manually mixing the spinach into the sauce with a wooden spoon!). For the pizza you may also want a baking stone. These are made of stone or ceramic and the crust tastes better than baking on a foil tray. Think of stone-baked pizza flavor versus other ovens. For any fish lovers out there, it's like the superior flavor of eating cedar-planked fish...

Notice in the shopping list there is a whole section for busy cooks titled "Food when you don't have time to cook." These items are all healthy, cost-effective, tasty, and satiating, in contrast with toxic fast food items. When I started cooking plant-based six years ago, I quickly found some meals required more prep time, like the legumes example in the Introduction. Busy people starting this transition may want to use some of these quick and easy options to take breaks

11

from plant-based cooking. No doubt many others have noticed they can fill up on corn chips and salsa. When you think about it, that's a complete plant-based meal of whole grain and vegetables: corn, tomato, onion, spices, and peppers. It always works in a time crunch and it's not going to break the bank. Neither does legumes with vegetables, e.g. roasted garlic hummus with pita chips and raw vegetables, but these are just break-glass-in-case-of-emergency quick and easy meals.

To discover more exciting, savory, plant-based meals you're ready to move on to Chapter 2. Inside, you'll discover a plethora of fast, kitchen-tested, savory meal options from all over the globe.

Chapter 2
Sample Meals

"Replace refined carbs with fruits, vegetables, whole grains and legumes like beans, hummus, tofu... for anti-cancer, anti-heart disease, and anti-aging properties."

- Dr. Dean Ornish, President of The Preventive Medicine Research Institute

Breakfast is optional!

Breakfast of Tofu Champions[11]

Serves 4 |Prep time: 10 min | Cook time: 8 min | Total 18 min

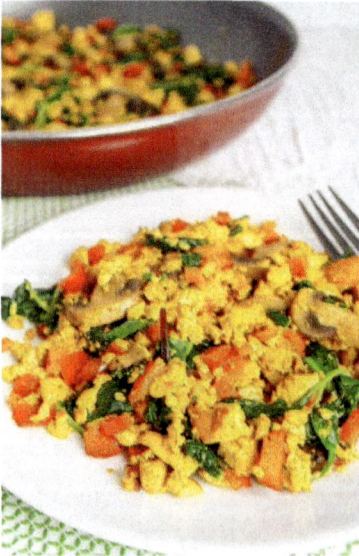

---

[11] Turnbull, S. (2022, February 22). *Tofu Scramble: Breakfast of (vegan) Champions*. It Doesn't Taste Like Chicken. https://itdoesnttastelikechicken.com/tofu-scramble-breakfast-vegan-champions/

You Need:

Spice Mix:
- o   Garlic powder, .25 tsp
- o   Turmeric, .75 tsp
- o   Salt, 1 tsp
- o   Cumin, 1 tsp
- o   Chili powder, 1 tsp
- o   Nutritional yeast, 2 tbsp

Tofu:
- o   Rinsed black beans, 19 oz
- o   A large block of tofu
- o   Minced garlic, two cloves
- o   Chopped onion, .5
- o   Chopped red pepper
- o   Sliced button mushrooms, 8 oz
- o   Oil, 1 tbsp

Method:

1. Start out by combining the spices together and place them to the side until later.
2. Sauté the onion, garlic, pepper, and mushrooms on medium heat. Allow all of this to cook together for about eight minutes or until it starts to brown.
3. Break up the tofu and add it to the skillet. Mash around until it looks like scrambled eggs. Mix in the beans and the spice mixture. Cook for about five to eight minutes and enjoy.

Spinach Omelet[12]

Serves 1 | Prep time: 10 min | Cook time: 10 min | Total 20 min

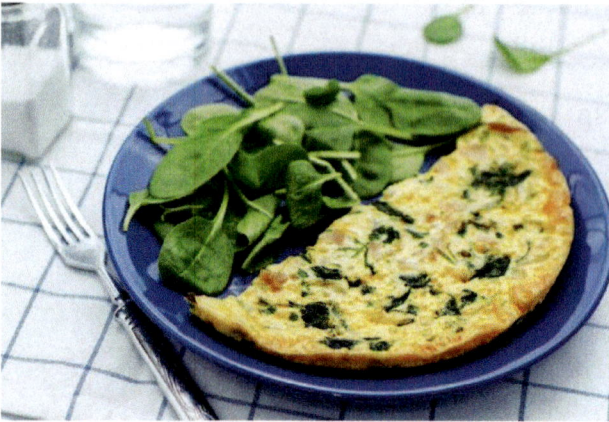

You Need:

- Pepper
- Salt
- Vegan butter, 2 tbsp
- Vegan cheese of choice, .33 c
- Spinach, 3 c
- Sliced mushrooms, e.g. Baby Bella, 1 c
- Minced garlic, one clove
- Vegan eggs, 2.5, e.g. Just Egg

Method:

1. Place the vegan butter and garlic into a skillet and add salt. Cook until fragrant and mix in the mushrooms. Cook until browned. Add spinach and cook until wilted. Put into a bowl and wipe the skillet out with a paper towel.
2. Beat vegan eggs together with pepper and salt. Add more vegan butter to the pan and pour in the eggs.

---

[12] Adapted from Chef, T. (2019, May 26). *Spinach Omelette*. The Take It Easy Chef. https://www.thetakeiteasychef.com/spinach-omelette-recipe

Rotate the pan around so that the eggs cover the pan. Once the egg has almost cooked through, add the cooked mushrooms and spinach to the eggs and all cheese. Fold the egg in half and enjoy.

Gingerbread Waffles[13]

Serves 6 | Prep time: 10 min | Cook time: 15 min | Total 25 min

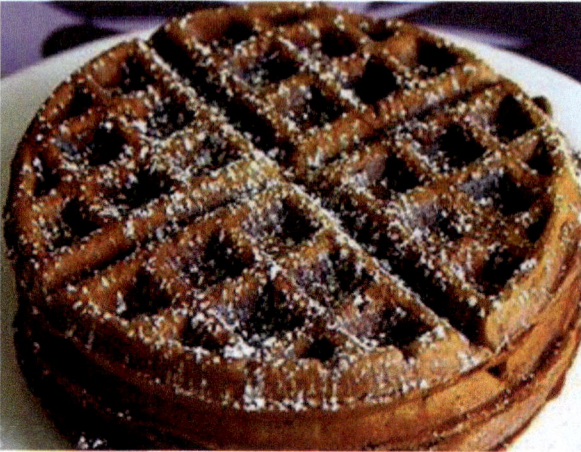

You Need:

- o Coconut sugar, 4 tbsp
- o Ground ginger, 2 tsp
- o Cinnamon, 1.5 tsp
- o Salt, .25 tsp
- o Baking soda, .25 tsp
- o Ground flax seeds, 1 tbsp
- o Spelt Flour, 1 c
- o Baking powder, 2 tsp
- o Olive oil, 1.5 tbsp
- o Molasses, 2 tbsp
- o Apple cider vinegar, 1 tbsp
- o Coconut milk, 1 c
- o Maple syrup to taste
- o Optional: powdered sugar

---

[13] Adapted from Dana @ Minimalist Baker. (n.d.). *waffles Archives*. Minimalist Baker. Vegan Gingerbread Waffles | Minimalist Baker Recipes

Method:

1. Start off by getting your waffle iron heated up, and then brush it with some oil.
2. If you don't feel like using your waffle iron, or if you don't have one, feel free to fix these as a pancake.
3. Mix the dry ingredients together. Stir together the wet ingredients. Now, mix everything together until just combined. It should be about the consistency of the cake batter. If it's too thick, add a little more milk.
4. Once the waffle iron is hot, pour in the batter and let them cook according to the instructions of your device.
5. Remove the waffles and continue with the rest of the batter. You may garnish with powdered sugar and maple syrup. Enjoy.

Smoothies

Peanut dream smoothie[14]

Serves 1 | Prep time: 5 min

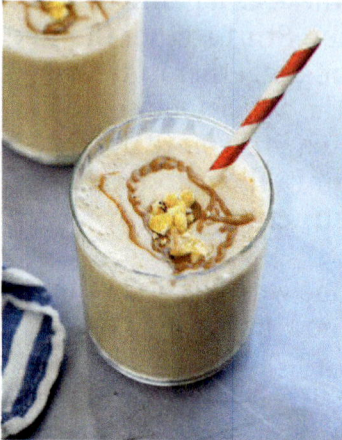

Ingredients:

- 1 cup unsweetened almond milk
- 1 frozen banana
- 1/2 cup pineapple
- 2 tablespoons naturalpeanut butter
- 2 tablespoons maca root powder (optional plant protein) or try pea protein powder post-workout!
- 1 cup ice

Directions:

Blend all ingredients until smooth. May garnish with pineapple tidbits.

---

[14]*The Peanut Butter Dream Smoothie! - Candice Kumai.* (n.d.). https://candicekumai.com/the-peanut-butter-booster-smoothie/

Chocolate Peanut Butter Banana Smoothie[15]

Serves 1 | Prep time: 5 min

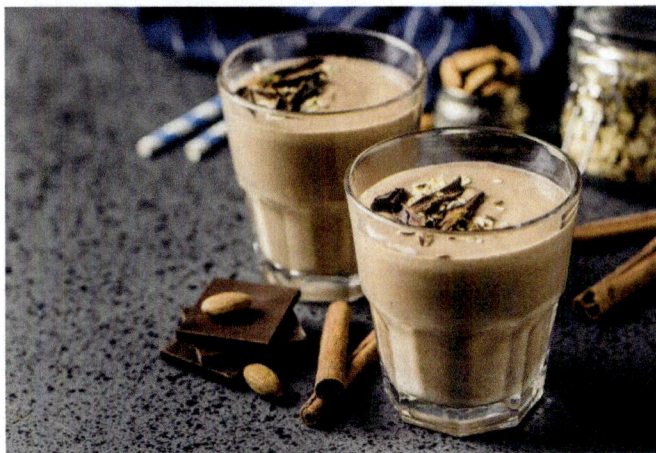

Ingredients

- o   2 whole, ripe bananas
- o   3 to 4 tablespoons cocoa powder
- o   1 tablespoon pure maple syrup
- o   1/4 cup peanut butter (I use Skippy Natural Creamy)
- o   3 cups vanilla almond milk/ vanilla coconut milk
- o   1/2 cup ice cubes

Method

1. Blend bananas with cocoa powder, maple syrup, and peanut butter. Process until mashed.
2. Add the almond milk and ice, blending until smooth.
3. May garnish with shredded dark dairy-free chocolate. This could be a meal replacement if you are in a time crunch.

---

[15]*The Best Vegan Chocolate Peanut Butter Banana Smoothie*. (2022, July 6). The Spruce Eats. https://www.thespruceeats.com/vegan-chocolate-peanut-butter-banana-smoothie-1000994

Nutrition Facts (per serving): 498 cal, 71g carbs, 21g fat, 12g protein

Remember the human body runs on sugar (see Chapter 1 in Book 1). Notice plant-based foods are rich in carbs. This aligns with Dr. Longo's recommendation on how to eat for long life based on interviewing hundreds of people living past 100: a high carb, low protein, plant-based diet.

Super Green Smoothie[16]

Serves 1 | Prep time: 5 min

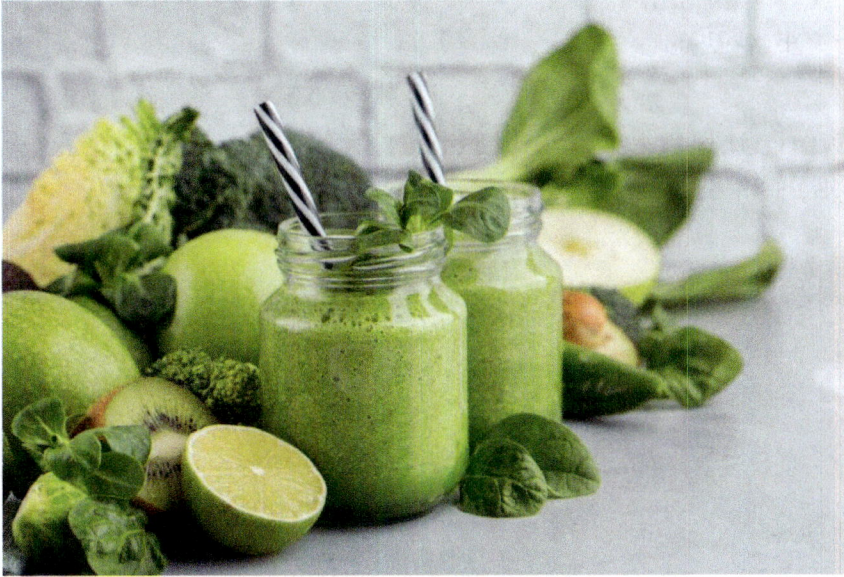

Ingredients:

- Ice cubes, 6 to 8
- Chia seeds, 1 tbsp
- Spinach, 2 c
- Ginger, small knob
- Carrots, 2
- Celery, two sticks
- Kale, two leaves

Method:

1. If your juicer has a low setting, set it to that first and juice the kale first. Then you can switch to the high setting and juice the ginger, carrots, and celery.

---

[16] Inspired by *A Rejuvenating Green Smoothie You Won't Be Able to Get Enough of.* (2021, May 12). The Spruce Eats.
https://www.thespruceeats.com/raw-food-green-kale-smoothie-3377470

2. Add the juice to the blender along with the ice, chia seeds, and spinach.
3. Mix until everything has come together and becomes smooth.
4. Enjoy

Nutrition Facts (per serving): 155 cal, 37g carbs, 1g fat, 3g protein

Blueberry Smoothie Bowl[17]

Serves 1 | Prep time: 5 min

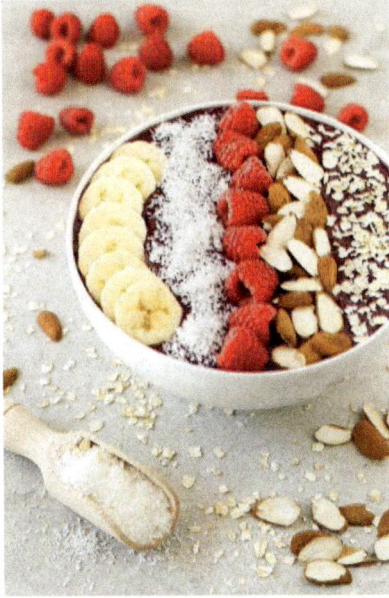

Ingredients:

- Unsweetened shredded coconut, 1 tbsp
- Sliced banana, .5
- Vanilla, 1 tsp
- Cashew butter, 1 tbsp
- Water, 2 tbsp
- Banana, .5
- Sliced almonds, 1 tbsp
- Frozen blueberries, 1 c
- Optional: raspberries or blackberries for topping

Method:

1. Add the vanilla, cashew butter, water, ½ of a banana, and blueberries into a blender and combine

---

[17] Adapted from *Blueberry Smoothie Bowl*. (2022, November 14). Simple Vegan Blog. https://simpleveganblog.com/blueberry-smoothie-bowl/

everything until it creates a smooth drink. Pour this into a bowl.

2. Top with the coconut, almonds, and sliced banana.

Nutrition Facts (½ the bowl): 556 cal, 102g carbs, 18g fat, 7.8g protein, 15.3g fiber - your daily dose of fiber in one bowl! The whole bowl is a full meal!

Please note if you would like nutrition info for any other recipes, you may find it in the online recipes. What's most important is consuming the daily serving sizes of each whole food. Remember from the Introduction that you do not have to count carbs or calories when eating whole foods, plant-based!

Salads and Bowls

Arugula Quinoa Bowl[18]

Serves 1 | Prep time: 10 min | Cook time: 15 min | Total 15 min

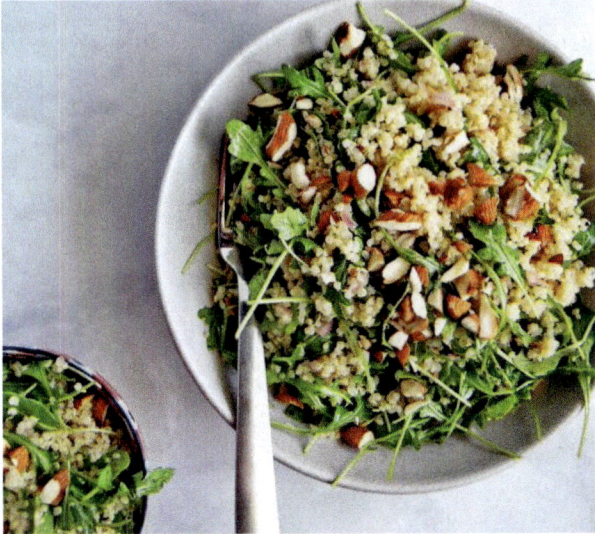

Ingredients:

- ○ Pepper
- ○ Salt
- ○ Crumbled vegan cheese, 2 tsp, e.g. vegan parmesan
- ○ Sherry vinegar, 1 tbsp
- ○ Chopped walnuts, 2 tbsp
- ○ Olive oil, 2 tsp
- ○ Chopped peaches, .25 c (optional - better to eat 10 min before rest of salad)
- ○ Arugula, 1 c
- ○ Sliced avocado, .5
- ○ Cooked quinoa, .75 c

---

[18]*Best Quinoa Arugula Salad with Lemon Vinaigrette*. (2022, June 28). My Everyday Table. https://myeverydaytable.com/quinoa-arugula-salad-with-lemon-vinaigrette/

  o lemon vinaigrette dressing

Method:

1. Put quinoa in boiling water, reduce heat and simmer for 15min until water absorbed
2. Whisk together pepper, salt, oil, and vinegar in a small bowl.
3. Put the arugula into the bottom of a medium bowl. Place the walnuts, peaches, avocados, and quinoa around the sides of the bowl. Drizzle dressing over and sprinkle on cheese.

Quinoa Salad[19]

Serves 6 | Prep Time: 10 min | Cook time: 15 min | Total 25 min

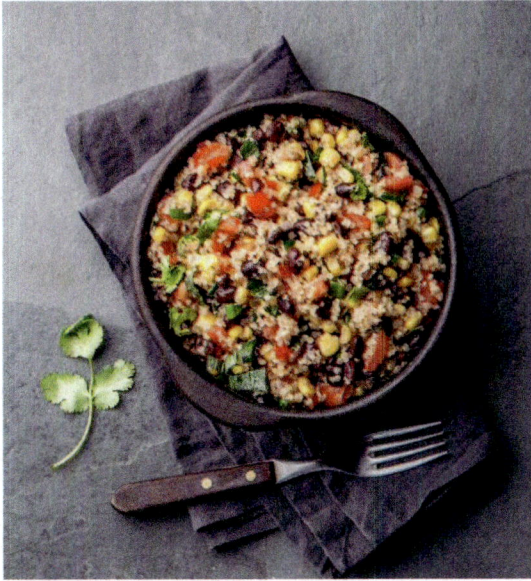

You Need:

- Pepper
- Salt
- Basil, six leaves
- Chopped tomato, 1 c
- Chopped bell pepper, 1 c
- Chopped spinach, 1 c
- Corn, 1.5 c
- Water, 1.5 c
- Dry quinoa, 1 c
- Dressing: lemon or balsamic vinaigrette
- Pepper, .25 tsp
- Salt, .25 tsp
- Chopped green onion, 1 tbsp

---

[19]*Favorite Quinoa Salad*. (2021, August 25). Cookie and Kate.
https://cookieandkate.com/best-quinoa-salad-recipe/

- Minced garlic clove
- Lemon zest, .25 tsp
- Juice of ½ lemon
- Orange juice, 1 tbsp
- Avocado oil, 2 tbsp

Method:

1. Clean your quinoa and then place them into a pot. Stir and toast the quinoa to remove any of the water that may still be on them from the rinsing process. Place the water into it and allow this to boil. Lower the heat so that it simmers for 13 minutes with the lid covering it.
2. As the quinoa cooks, mix all of the dressing ingredients together.
3. Chop all the vegetables.
4. When the quinoa is cooked, fluff it, and add some pepper and salt. Mix in the veggies, dressing, and some fresh basil.

Ancient Grains Bowl (from True Food Kitchen)[20]

Serves 2 | Prep time: 10 min | Cook time: 40 min | Total 50 min

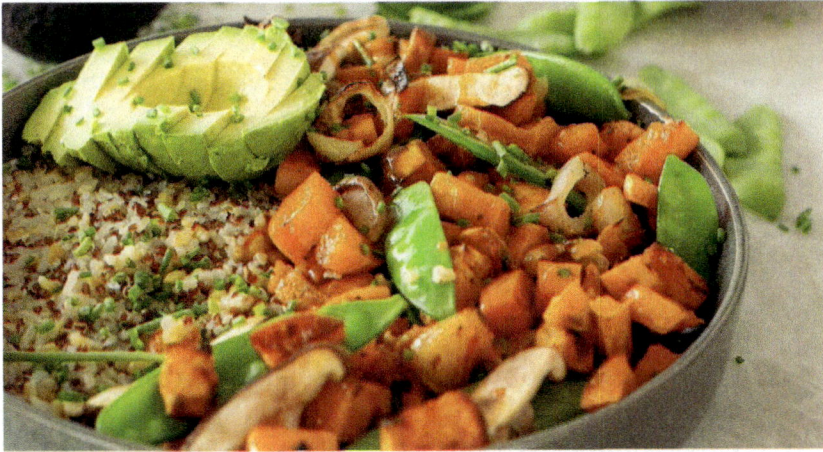

You Need:

- o 2 sweet potatoes, peeled and diced
- o 1 small red onion, peeled and sliced
- o 1-2 tablespoons extra virgin olive oil
- o sea salt and pepper to taste
- o 2 servings ancient grains of your choice, cooked to package instructions, e.g. barley, millet, sorghum. You can also use multicolor quinoa (cooks in 15min)
- o 1 1/2 tablespoons honey
- o 1 tablespoon Sambal Oelek (add more or less depending on how you like the heat!
- o 1 tablespoon Dijon mustard
- o 1/2 cup snow peas
- o ¾ cup mushrooms, sliced
- o 1 ripe avocado, sliced

[20] Spiker, L. (2020, October 21). *Copycat True Food Kitchen Ancient Grains Bowl!* The Organic Kitchen Blog and Tutorials. https://www.theorganickitchen.org/copycat-true-food-kitchen-ancient-grains-bowl/

- 1 tablespoon chives for garnish
- Optional: pesto sauce (If you don't want to make your own, you could buy at Trader Joe's)

Method:

1. Preheat oven to 425°F, line rimmed cookie sheet with parchment paper, set aside
2. Add potatoes and onion, drizzle with olive oil, sprinkle with sea salt and freshly ground pepper, toss.
3. Bake in oven 35 minutes
4. Cook grains ~20-40min depending on grains on hand.
5. While grains cook, slice chives and mushrooms. Whisk together honey, sambal oelek, and dijon mustard, set aside
6. When potatoes are almost done (crispy browned) add mushrooms and snow peas to the pan and set timer for 5 more minutes.
7. Divide cooked grains into two bowls, top with veggies, drizzle with sauce from step 5, leaving some in a small bowl to use as needed. Add avocado, chives. Add pesto if using. Enjoy!

Quinoa Gado-Gado Bowl[21]

Serves 2 | Prep time: 10 min | Cook time: 20 min | Total 30 min

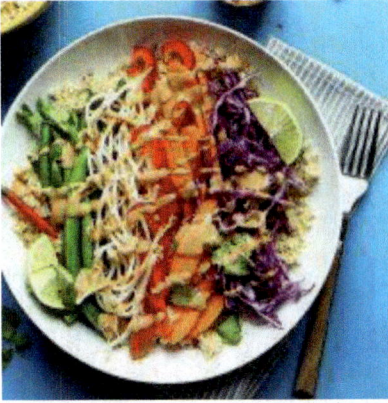

You Need:

For Spicy Peanut Sauce:
- Water, 3 – 4 tbsp
- Creamy peanut butter, .33 c
- Chili garlic sauce, 1 tsp
- Soy sauce, 1 tbsp
- Lime juice, 3 tbsp
- Maple syrup, 2 – 3 tbsp

For Gado-Gado:
- Thinly sliced carrots, 2
- Quinoa, .5 c
- Thinly shredded red cabbage, .66 c
- Water, 1 c
- Mung bean sprouts, .75 c
- Trimmed green beans, 1 c
- Thinly sliced red bell pepper, .5

---

[21] Dana @ Minimalist Baker. (2020, July 15). *Quinoa Gado-Gado Bowl (30 Minutes!)*. Minimalist Baker. https://minimalistbaker.com/quinoa-gado-gado-bowl-30-minutes/

Method:

1. Cook quinoa according to the directions on the package.
2. Steam the green beans while the quinoa is cooking. Once they are steamed, add them to ice water to stop them from cooking. Set to the side.
3. To make the peanut sauce: add the chili garlic sauce, peanut butter, maple syrup, lime juice, and soy sauce to a bowl and mix everything together. Add one tablespoon at a time until it makes a pourable sauce. You do not want this too thin.
4. Taste and adjust seasonings if needed.
5. To serve equally, divide quinoa into two bowls. Top with carrots, mung bean sprouts, red bell pepper, and green beans. Drizzle over the peanut sauce. Can garnish with a sprinkle of red pepper flakes, lime wedges, or cilantro, if desired.

Black Bean and Avocado Bowl[22]

Serves 1 | Prep time: 10 min | Cook time: 10 min | Total 20 min

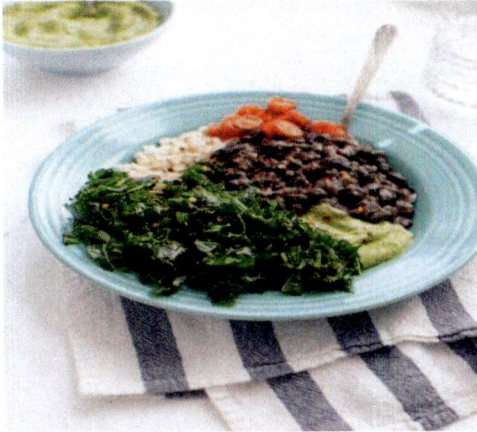

You Need:

- Pepper
- Cilantro leaves, 2 tbsp
- Salt
- Black beans, warmed, .5 c
- Olive oil, 1 tsp
- Thinly sliced medium radish, 1
- Grape tomatoes, .5 c
- Thinly slice avocado, .5
- Corn kernels from one ear

Method:

1. Add the beans into a shallow bowl and set to the side. Place a small skillet on medium heat. Add olive oil and allow to warm up. Place tomatoes into skillet and cook until charred. Shake the pan to turn the

---

[22] Inspired by Kate, K. (2017, December 3). *Kale, Black Bean & Avocado Burrito Bowl*. Cookie and Kate. https://cookieandkate.com/kale-black-bean-and-avocado-burrito-bowl/

tomatoes. Put the tomatoes beside the beans in a bowl.
2. Add corn to the skillet and heat through. Put the corn beside the tomatoes. Add cilantro, sliced radish, and sliced avocado to the bowl. Sprinkle on pepper and salt. Enjoy.

Tempeh Salad with Brussels Sprouts[23]

Serves 2 | Prep time: 10 min | Cook time: 10 min | Total 20 min

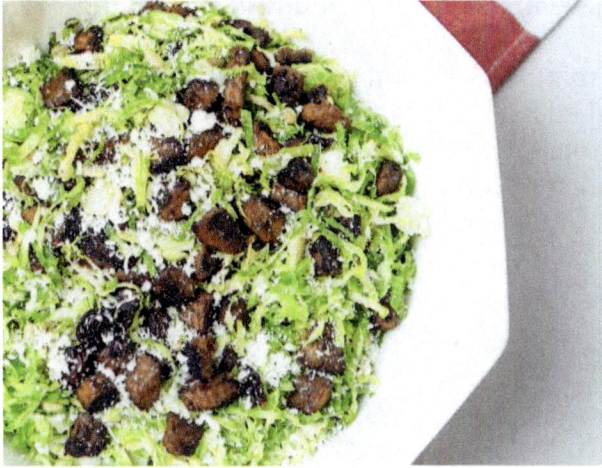

You Need:

- Lime wedges, 2
- Salt
- Sesame oil, 2 tbsp
- Chopped, toasted unsalted peanuts, 2 tbsp
- Chopped cilantro, 2 tbsp
- Thinly sliced tempeh, 4 oz
- Rice vinegar, 2 tsp
- Sliced Fresno chili, 6
- Low sodium soy sauce, 4 tsp
- Thinly sliced Brussels sprouts, 1.5 c

Method:

1. Place some of the oil into a skillet and let it start to heat up. Place in the tempeh and cook until it is

---

[23]*Brussels Sprouts and Crispy Tempeh With Soy Dressing.* (2018, December 5). Cooking Light. https://www.cookinglight.com/recipes/brussels-sprouts-and-crispy-tempeh-with-soy-dressing

browned and crisp. Place on a plate and set to the side.

2. Add a tablespoon of cilantro, the rest of the sesame oil, salt, vinegar, and soy sauce, and mix it all together. Place in the sprouts and toss everything together.

3. Divide this mixture between two bowls. Top with the peanuts and sliced Chile, and then place the crispy tempeh on top. Drizzle the top with the remaining dressing and sprinkle with some extra cilantro.

4. Serve with a wedge of lime and enjoy.

Chickpea and Sweet Potato Salad[24]

Serves 4 | Prep time: 10 min | Cook time: 10 min | Total 20 min

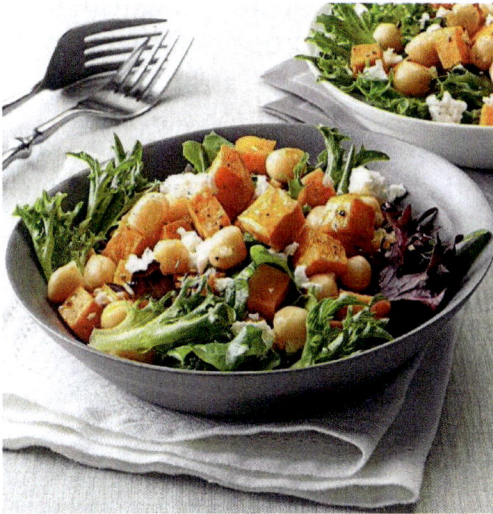

You Need:

- o Pepper
- o Salt
- o Baby arugula, 5 oz
- o Sweet potatoes, four small
- o Drained and rinsed chickpeas, 15 oz can
- o Almond butter, .25 c
- o Olive oil, 2 tbsp
- o Warm water, 3.5 tbsp
- o Lemon juice, 3 tbsp

Method:

1. Pierce the sweet potatoes all over with a fork. Put on a microwavable plate and cook in the microwave for

---

24 Based on Cochennec, G. L. (2019, June 10). *Sweet Potato And Chickpea Salad Recipe by Tasty*. tasty.co. https://tasty.co/recipe/sweet-potato-and-chickpea-salad

around five minutes. Carefully remove and slice into .5-inch-thick rounds.

2. Place lemon juice, water, and almond butter in a bowl and mix everything together. Set to the side

3. Brush the potato slices with oil. Heat up a pan and cook up some slices of potatoes. Cook potato slices until golden brown.

4. Add pepper, salt, two tablespoons juice, one tablespoon oil, arugula, and chickpeas in a large bowl. Toss everything together and then separate them out between four plates. Top with sweet potatoes and drizzle with almond butter sauce.

Corn and Black Bean Salad[25]

Serves 2 | Prep time: 5 min | Total 20min

You Need:

- Hot sauce, 1 tsp
- Ground cumin, 1 tsp
- Lime juice, 1 tbsp
- Chopped red onion, .5 c
- Rinsed black beans, 1 c
- Corn, 1 c
- Chopped red pepper
- Chopped cherry tomatoes, 1 c

Method:

This is an easy recipe to fix. All you have to do is place everything in a bowl and stir it all together. Season as you would like, and let everything come together in the fridge for about 15 minutes.

---

[25]Veganista, S. T. J. |. (2021, May 31). *Black Bean, Corn & Avocado Salad*. THE SIMPLE VEGANISTA. https://simple-veganista.com/black-bean-roasted-corn-tomato-salad/

Pastas

Remember whole grain pasta for maximum health benefits!

Savory sausage pasta

Serves 2 | Cook time: 30 min | Total 30 min

A former chef requested this recipe. Enjoy!

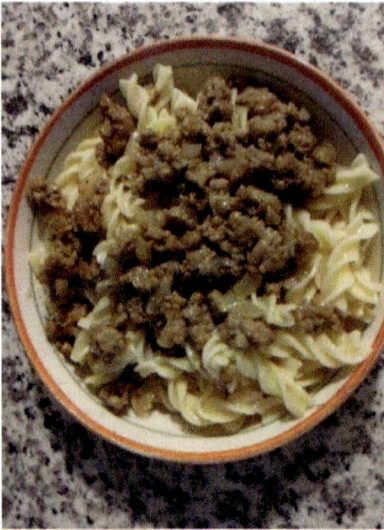

Ingredients:

- ½ Spanish or vidalia onion
- 1 tsp Minced garlic (1 clove)
- 1 lb ground plant sausage e.g. Impossible sausage savory
- Extra virgin olive oil, cold pressed (EVOO), enough to thinly coat pan
- ½ lb fusilli or penne pasta, whole grain recommended
- 1 can vegetable broth* (I use ½ tsp vegetable Better than Bouillon stirred in 1 cup water)
- Paprika and ground pepper

* The bouillon in water is much cheaper with less waste than buying pre-packed vegetable broth. It also tastes better.

Directions:

1. Brown sausage in EVOO, sprinkle with dash of paprika and ground pepper, dice onion, boil pasta
2. Drain sausage on paper towel, dump oil (may skip this step)
3. Add fresh EVOO, teaspoon minced garlic (1 clove)
4. Caramelize diced onion
5. Add sausage, pepper, and vegetable broth
6. Reduce heat from boil to simmer, add ground pepper if you want more bite

Vegan Lasagna[26]

Serves 9 | Prep time: 35 min | Cook time: 30 min | Total 1 hr 5 min

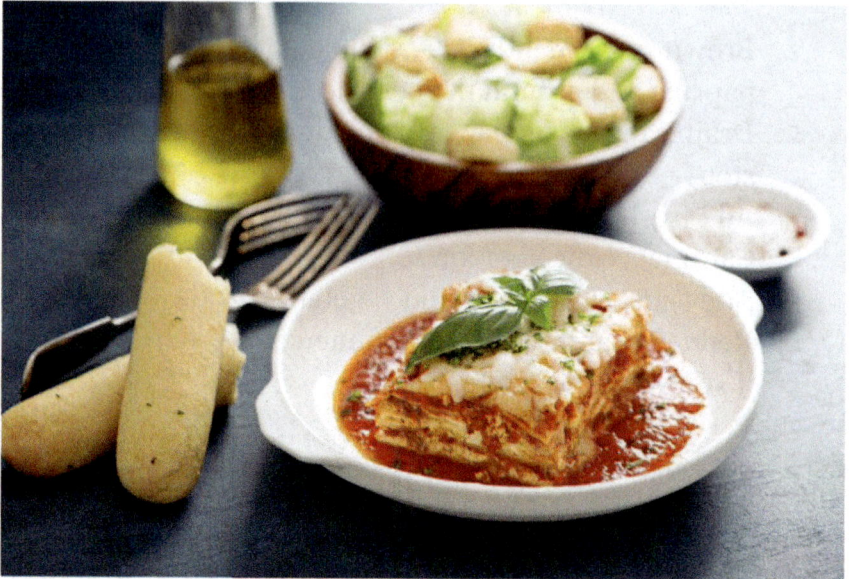

You Need:

Cashew cream:
- o Dijon, .5 tsp
- o Sea salt, .75 tsp
- o Apple cider vinegar, 2 tsp
- o Lemon juice, 2 tbsp
- o Water, 1 c
- o Raw cashews, 2 c – soak for four hours if you don't have a high-powered blender

Vegetables:
- o Minced garlic, two cloves
- o Baby spinach, 5 to 6 oz – chopped
- o Pepper

[26] Adapted from Hylton, J. (2021, July 6). *The Best Vegan Lasagna.* Jessica in the Kitchen. https://jessicainthekitchen.com/best-vegan-lasagna-recipe/

- Sea salt, .5 tsp
- Baby Bella mushrooms, 8 oz – chopped
- Chopped onion, one large
- EVOO, 2 tbsp

Everything else:
- Vegan parmesan and vegan mozzarella
- No-boil lasagna noodles, 9
- Marinara sauce, 2.5 c

Method:

1. Set your oven to 425. Soak and rinse the cashews until they run clear.
2. In a blender, add the mustard, salt, vinegar, lemon juice, water, and cashews. Combine until creamy and smooth. If the mixture is thick, slowly add in additional water until it smooths out.
3. Add oil to a skillet and cook the mushrooms and onions with some pepper and salt. Cook for about eight to ten minutes.
4. Slowly add in the spinach, letting each additional wilt down before adding more. Add the garlic, cooking until fragrant. Add more pepper and salt.
5. Add ¾ of a cup of sauce to the bottom of a square baking dish. Place three noodles and top with a cup of cashew cream. Top with half of the veggies. Add another ¾ cup of tomato sauce. Top with three more noodles and another cup of cream. Add in the remaining veggies. Place the last three noodles on and cover with ¾ cup of sauce and top with mozzarella.
6. Wrap with foil or parchment paper. Bake for 25 minutes. Rotate the pan and cook for another five to ten minutes.
7. Let the lasagna rest for 15 to 20 minutes. Drizzle the remaining cashew cream over the top and sprinkle with basil. Optional: add parmesan to taste.

Vegan Spicy Sausage Pasta[27]

Serves 6 | Prep time: 15 min | Cook time: 10 min | Total 25 min

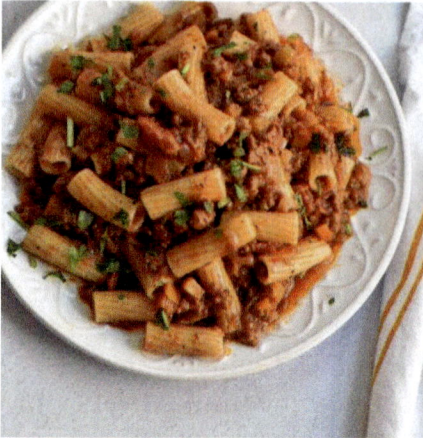

You Need:

- Pepper and salt
- vegan parmesan, 1 c
- Full-fat oat milk, 1 c
- Vegetable stock, .5 c
- White wine, .25 c
- Bunch of baby broccoli florets
- Sun-dried tomato in oil, 4 tbsp – chopped
- Sliced garlic, six cloves
- Impossible Sausage, 14 oz – spicy
- Canola or olive oil, 1 tbsp
- 16 oz pasta

Method:

1. Boil pasta
2. Brown sausage in oil. Remove sausage to drain on paper towels.

---

[27] Jeni. (2021, September 29). *Spicy Vegan Sausage Pasta*. Thyme & Love. https://thymeandlove.com/spicy-vegan-sausage-pasta/

3. In the same pan, add the broccoli, tomatoes, and garlic. Cook for a minute and remove from heat.
4. Deglaze the pan with the wine and heat for about a minute. Add in the oat milk and stock, cooking for two minutes or until it starts to reduce.
5. Stir the broccoli, pasta, and cheese into the sauce. Add in the sausage and cook for another minute.
6. Season with pepper and salt, and enjoy.

I'd love to hear from you!

If you find any of these tips or recipes helpful or just love a particular recipe, please share by leaving a review on Amazon:

https://www.amazon.com/review/create-review/?ie&asin=B0C87DH21W

It's through your support and reviews this book can help more people. Your review could help someone you know live healthy, long and strong. It may also help someone struggling to prepare fast, flavorful, filling recipes. Your valuable feedback will also help me with future editions and upcoming books in this series.

Thank you for reading!

Spaghetti with Beyond Meatballs[28]

Serves 4 | Prep time: 20 min | Cook time: 35 min | Total 55 min

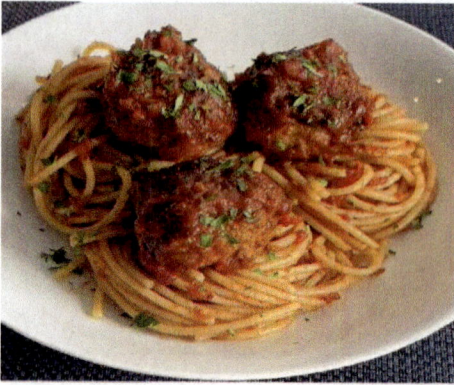

You Need:

- o Dried parsley, 1.5 tsp
- o Vegan breadcrumbs, 1 tbsp
- o Beyond Meat Ground, 1 lb.
- o Pepper, .5 tsp - divided
- o Salt, 1.25 tsp – divided
- o Oregano, 1 tsp
- o Tomato sauce, 8 oz
- o Minced garlic, three cloves
- o Chopped medium onion
- o Olive oil, 4 tbsp – divide
- o Diced tomatoes, 28 oz can – drained, juice reserved
- o Spaghetti, 12 oz
- o Onion powder, .25 tsp
- o Garlic powder, .25 tsp

---

[28]*Vegan Spaghetti and (Beyond) Meatballs*. (2022, June 16). Allrecipes. https://www.allrecipes.com/recipe/278805/vegan-spaghetti-and-beyond-meatballs/

Method:

1. Add two tablespoons of the oil to a pot with the garlic and onion. Cook for about two minutes, stirring. Add in the tomatoes and their juice, a quarter teaspoon of pepper, half a teaspoon of salt, oregano, and tomato sauce. Let this come up to a simmer, and let it cook as you fix the meatballs.
2. Combine the vegan meat with the onion powder, garlic powder, remaining pepper, remaining salt, parsley, and breadcrumbs. Once mixed together, roll them into one-and-a-half-inch balls.
3. Add slightly salted water to a pot and let it boil. Add in the spaghetti, cooking for 12 minutes.
4. Meanwhile, add the rest of the oil to a skillet and cook the meatballs. Turn them occasionally, cooking for about ten minutes.
5. Pour the sauce over the meatballs and mix. Simmer for an additional ten minutes.
6. Serve spaghetti topped with sauce and meatballs.

Creamy mushroom risotto[29]

Serves 4 | Prep time: 10 min | Cook time: 35 min | Total 45 min

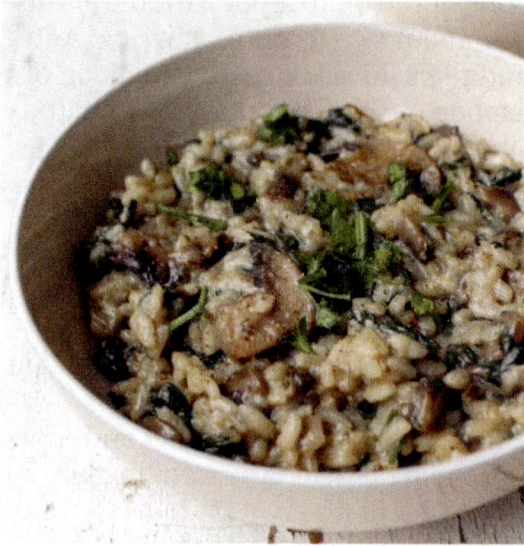

Ingredients:

- o 1 Tbsp Olive Oil
- o 1 Medium Vidalia onion, chopped
- o 5 cups (480g) Cremini Mushrooms sliced or 5 asparagus stalks chopped
- o 1 Tbsp Crushed Garlic (1 clove)
- o 1 and ½ cups (300g) Arborio Rice - may use brown for max health, but it will change the flavor
- o 6 cups Vegetable Stock Divided (I prefer 3 tsp vegetable Better than Bouillon mixed in 3 cups water for a more savory outcome)
- o 2 tbsp vegan butter
- o Sea salt and ground black pepper to taste

---

[29]Based on Andrews, A. (2021, September 8). *Creamy Vegan Mushroom Risotto*. Loving It Vegan. https://lovingitvegan.com/creamy-vegan-mushroom-risotto/

Instructions:

1. Sauté chopped onion on medium high for a couple of minutes until soft.
2. Add sliced mushrooms and garlic
3. Cook for 2 minutes until the mushrooms have released some of their water.
4. Add rice and sauté it with the onions, mushrooms, and garlic.
5. Add 3 cups vegetable stock, stir, simmer for around 20 minutes until the broth is mostly absorbed. *Add asparagus with broth if not using mushrooms
6. Add 1½ cups vegetable stock, stir and simmer ~10 minutes until the broth is mostly absorbed.
7. Add remaining stock, stir and simmer for a final 5-10 minutes.
8. Mix in the butter.
9. Add sea salt to taste.
10. Serve with fresh ground black pepper.

Polish Inspired

Vegan haluski - polish comfort food[30]

Serves 3 | Prep time: 15 min | Cook time: 30 min | Total 45 min

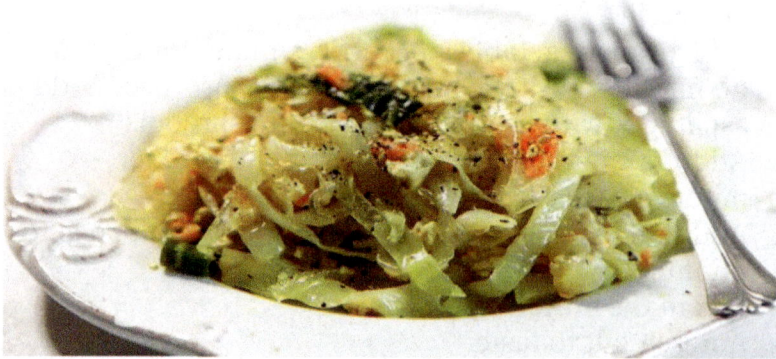

Ingredients:

- 2 tbsp canola oil or olive oil, cold-pressed
- 1 large sweet onion
- 6 cups shredded cabbage (about 1 small head, red or green)
- 1/2 tsp garlic powder
- 1/4 tsp turmeric (optional)
- sea salt to taste, fresh ground pepper to taste
- 1 block firm tofu (1lb/450g) (optional, will serve 2 without it)
- 16oz rice noodles (international aisle with thai food packets)
- 1/4 cup vegan butter, e.g. Earth Balance

---

[30] Adapted from *Vegan Haluski – Cabbage and Noodles – Vegan Easy.* (2020, January 16). veganeasy.org.
https://www.veganeasy.org/recipes/vegan-haluski-cabbage-and-noodles/

Method:

1. Boil the noodles
2. Slice onion in long thin slices.
3. In a large pot cook the onion in oil, low heat for about 8 minutes
4. Cut the cabbage into ⅛" wide slices.
5. Add the cabbage, sprinkle with salt and pepper, and increase heat to medium.
6. Crumble in drained tofu if desired
7. Add garlic powder, turmeric, salt, and pepper and cook for about 15 minutes stirring frequently until cabbage wilts down and loses its bright color.
8. Add the noodles and butter coating all noodles and veggies, cook 1 minute.
9. Add salt and fresh ground pepper to taste. Enjoy!

American Inspired

Chef special! Mom's herb-crusted meatloaf

Serves 3 | Prep time: 15 min | Cook time: 30 min | Total 45 min

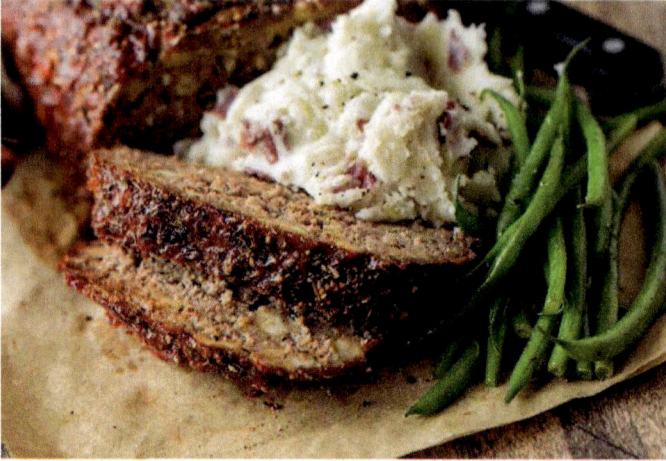

Ingredients:

- 1 lb Beyond Meat plant-based ground
- 1 tsp minced garlic (1 clove in garlic press)
- 1/2 vidalia onion diced
- 5 tbsp Marinara sauce
- 1 tbsp each of sage, basil, rosemary
- 1 cup brown precooked rice
- 2 tbsp sea salt
- 2 tbsp olive or canola oil
- Optional: a few small potatoes and carrots cut up in quarters with the same spices; arrange on foil around the loaf, then drizzle olive oil lightly on potatoes and carrots only. Note potatoes and carrots have to be pre boiled for 5 minutes and cooled.

Directions:

1. Preheat oven to 400°F, boil pot of water
2. Sauté onion and garlic in olive oil until golden, drain off most of the oil but leave a little
3. While caramelizing onion, in a medium mixing bowl use a wooden spatula to poke holes into plant ground. Mix in herbs and marinara
4. Add drained onions and garlic, mix all together.
5. Once blended form into loaf or football shape on foil lined pan
6. Then add a little marinara over top of the loaf, tent with foil but be sure it doesn't stick to the loaf. So it's tight around the edges but elevated on the top.
7. Bake 30min
8. Add rice to pot, stir in 1 tsp vegetable Bouillon, and simmer on medium until water absorbed, ~15min
9. Plate strips of loaf on a bed of rice, season to taste with sea salt. May also season rice with your preferred seasoning (I like Mrs. Dash Tomato, Basil & Garlic).

Mexican Inspired

Mexican bean salad[31]

Serves 4 | Prep time 15 min | Total time 45 min

This is a super easy, fast, tasty, healthy lunch for busy people. Buying the ingredients takes longer than the meal prep!

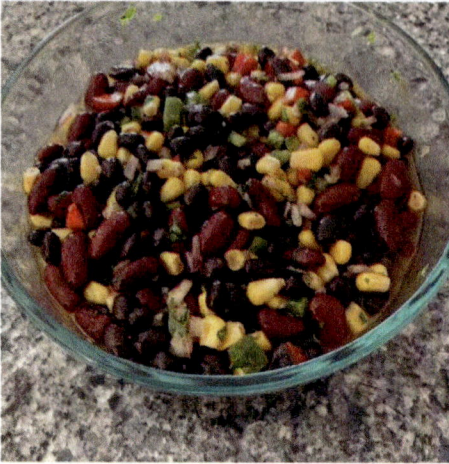

Ingredients:

- 1 (15 ounce) can black beans, rinsed and drained
- 1 (15 ounce) can red kidney beans, rinsed and drained
- 1 (15 ounce) can cannellini beans, rinsed and drained
- 1 green bell pepper, chopped
- 1 red bell pepper, chopped
- 1 (10 ounce) package frozen corn kernels, thawed
- 1 red onion, diced
- ½ cup olive oil
- ½ cup red wine vinegar

---

[31] Adapted from *Mexican Bean Salad*. (2022, August 22). Allrecipes. https://www.allrecipes.com/recipe/14169/mexican-bean-salad/

- ¼ cup chopped fresh cilantro
- 2 tablespoons fresh lime juice
- 1 tablespoon lemon juice
- 1 clove garlic, crushed
- 2 tablespoons white sugar
- 1 tablespoon salt
- 1 ½ teaspoons ground cumin
- 1 ½ teaspoons ground black pepper
- ½ teaspoon chili powder, or to taste
- 1 dash hot pepper sauce (optional)

Directions:

1. Mix beans, bell peppers, corn, and red onion in a large bowl.
2. Make dressing: whisk together remaining ingredients in a mixing bowl. Season with chili powder and hot sauce if desired.
3. Pour dressing over bean mixture and toss well. Refrigerate for 30-45min (until corn is thawed). Serve cold.

Vegan Enchilada Skillet[32]

Serves 6 | Prep time: 5 mins | Cook time: 25 mins | Total 30 mins

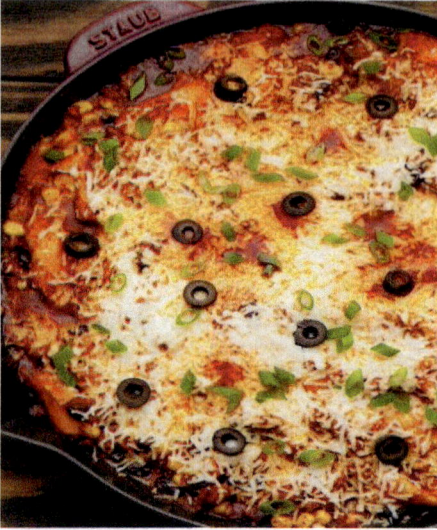

You Need:

- Pepper
- Salt
- Avocado, 1
- Oil, 2 tbsp
- Diced green onions, 2
- Sliced corn tortillas, 10
- Diced jalapeno, 1 (optional)
- Diced red onion, .5
- Chopped cilantro, a bunch
- Minced garlic, three cloves
- Chopped kale leaves, 4
- Peeled and cubed small butternut squash, 1
- Enchilada sauce, 10 oz
- Chili powder, 1.5 tsp
- Crushed tomatoes, 1 c

---

[32] McMinn, S. (2020, July 13). *Vegan Enchiladas Skillet*. My Darling Vegan. https://www.mydarlingvegan.com/vegan-skillet-enchiladas/

- o Cumin, .5 tsp
- o Whole kernel corn, .5 c
- o Paprika, .5 tsp
- o Black beans, one can

Method:

1. Put one tablespoon of oil into a hot pan. When heated, place in the tortilla strips and cook until crispy and brown. Allow this to drain on some paper towels.
2. Pour the rest of the oil, add onions, and let everything cook until they have softened and start to smell. Then add the garlic.
3. Add salt, paprika, cumin, chili powder, and butternut squash. Stir to coat with spices and lower heat, and cover. Allow this all to cook until the squash has become tender.
4. Add kale, enchilada sauce, tomatoes, corn, and black beans. Cook for three more minutes or until the kale has wilted. Give this a taste and add in some seasonings to taste.
5. Stir in tortillas and simmer for ten minutes until the liquid has mostly been absorbed. Take off the eye and let it sit for ten minutes before serving.
6. Garnish with green onions, cilantro, and jalapeno.

Bean and Tomato Casserole[33]

Serves 6 | Prep time: 10 min | Cook time: 35 min | Total 45 min

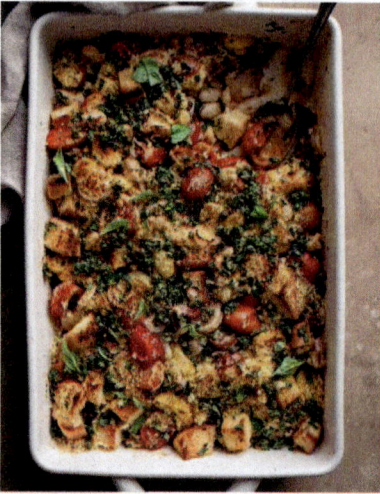

"This panzanella-inspired Tomato and White Bean Casserole is the perfect light lunch or dinner... It's bursting with fresh flavor from cherry tomatoes and shallots, mixed between layers of crunchy toasted bread, and topped with a cashew parmesan and a caper gremolata."

You Need:

- Black pepper
- 10 ounces (285g) of soft but sturdy rustic bread
- Extra virgin olive oil, 1½ tbsp
- Kosher salt
- 2 pounds (900g) cherry tomatoes or grape tomatoes, sliced in half
- 5 medium shallots (6-7 ounces or 170-200g), peeled and sliced into rings
- 4 garlic cloves, chopped

---

33 Nisha. (2022, February 17). *Tomato and White Bean Casserole*. Rainbow Plant Life. https://rainbowplantlife.com/tomato-and-white-bean-casserole/

- o 1 tablespoon fresh thyme leaves
- o 2 (15-ounce/425g) cans of cannellini beans, drained and rinsed
- o Freshly cracked black pepper

Cashew Parmesan
- o ½ cup (70g) raw cashews
- o 2 tablespoons nutritional yeast
- o ½ teaspoon kosher salt
- o ½ teaspoon extra virgin olive oil

Caper Gremolata
- o ¾cup(9g) Italian flat-leaf parsley leaves
- o ½cup(7-8g) fresh basil leaves
- o 2large garlic cloves, left whole and peeled
- o 2tablespoonscapers, drained
- o Flaky or coarse sea salt

Method:

1. Preheat the oven to 350°F. Chop the bread into ¾-inch cubes and transfer to a baking sheet. Drizzle with oil and salt. Bake for 10 minutes to lightly golden.

2. While baking bread, in your largest mixing bowl add tomatoes and shallots. Separate the shallots into individual rings as best you can. Add garlic, thyme, and beans. Drizzle 2 tbsp of oil, 1 ½ teaspoons of kosher salt and lots of fresh black pepper. Toss.

3. Add the baked bread cubes and gently toss to ensure the bread cubes are coated. Transfer the tomato mixture to a 3-quart/3-liter baking dish.

4. Bake the casserole 35-40 minutes, until the top bread pieces are crunchy.

5. Prep the Cashew Parmesan. Add the cashews, nutritional yeast, 1/2 tsp kosher salt, and 1/2 tsp oil to

a food processor. Pulse repeatedly to a fine, crumbly texture (like grated parmesan). Note: if you continuously blend you'll end up with cashew butter (a welcome, healthy spread you could add to any lunch bowl).

6. Prep Caper Gremolata. Give parsley and basil a fine chop. Add minced garlic. Top with capers and chop everything together. Sprinkle with coarse sea salt.

7. Sprinkle some coarse sea salt. Remove the casserole. Using oven mitts, arrange an oven rack for the broiler (but don't position it too close to the flame) and set your broiler to a low heat.

8. Add a generous layer of Cashew Parmesan on top of the baked dish and put it under the broiler for 1-2 minutes until the topping is nicely browned.

9. Cool for 10 minutes, then top with the Caper Gremolata. Finish with sprinkled olive oil and coarse sea salt. Enjoy!

Black Bean Burritos[34]

Serves 6 | Prep time: 10 min | Cook time: 15 min | Total 25 min

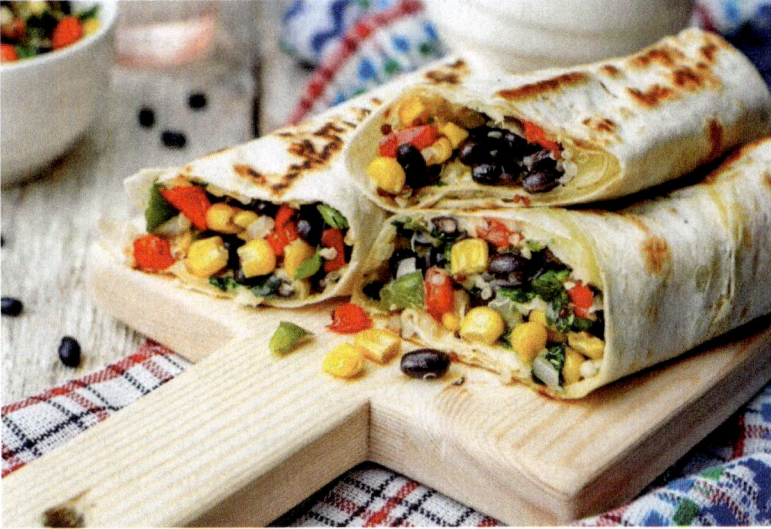

You Need:

For the Red Rice:
- o   Dry white rice, 1 c
- o   Water, .25 c
- o   Diced fresh tomato, 1 c
- o   Vegetable broth, 1 c
- o   Minced garlic, two cloves
- o   Diced white onion, 1 medium – reserve .25 cup
- o   Olive oil, 1 tbsp

For the Chili Lime Black Beans:
- o   Black beans, two cans – drained and rinsed
- o   Cumin, 2 tsp
- o   Chili powder, .75 tsp
- o   Pepper, 1 tsp
- o   Sea salt, 1 tsp

34 Marly, M. (2021, March 30). *Vegan Black Bean Burrito*. Namely Marly. https://namelymarly.com/vegan-black-bean-burrito/

- o Minced garlic, one clove
- o Lime juice, 2 tbsp

For Burritos:
- o Cilantro, .25 c per burrito
- o Guacamole, .25 c per burrito
- o Grated carrot, .25 c per burrito
- o Large corn tortillas

Method:

1. Cook the garlic and onion in some of the oil for about six to seven minutes until fragrant.
2. Add in the tomato, water, broth, and rice and cook, covered, until the rice is cooked through. This takes about 10 to 15 minutes.
3. Add in the reserved onion and garlic with the beans, pepper, chili powder, salt, cumin, and lime juice. With a potato masher, mash up some of the beans and cook for five to eight minutes until heated.
4. When the beans and rice are done, add to a large tortilla with your favorite toppings.

Caribbean Inspired

Cuban Black Bean Soup[35]

Serves 4 | Prep time: 30 min

This is a true gem based on a favorite dish at Bahama Breeze.

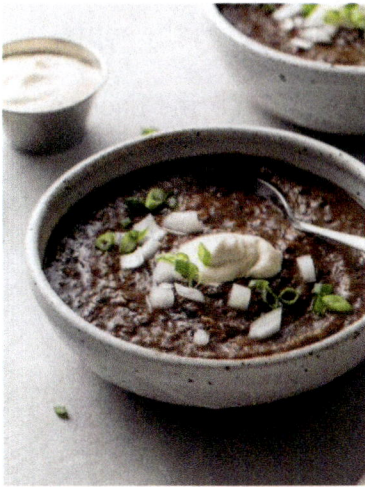

Ingredients:

- 4 cans (15 oz. each) Black Beans
- 1 Tbsp. Olive Oil
- 1 bottle (12 oz.) Beer
- ½ cup Water
- 1 Tbsp. Sherry, Dry
- ¾ cup Onions, diced
- ½ cup Green peppers, diced
- 2 Tbsp. Garlic
- ¼ tsp Ground Cumin
- 2 tsp Tabasco sauce
- To Taste Adobo seasoning, salt and pepper

---

[35] Adapted from https://www.bahamabreeze.com/recipe/appetizers-sides-soups-salads/black-bean-soup/prod2040224

Method:

1. Heat oil in a pot on medium heat.
2. Add the peppers, onions and garlic. Sauté for approximately 2 minutes.
3. Add the beer and Tabasco sauce, and bring to a boil.
4. Add 3 cans of beans with their juice and bring back to a boil.
5. Using a handheld kitchen blender, purée the soup until smooth.
6. Add the remaining 1 can of beans and bring back to a boil.
7. Add the Sherry wine, and season to taste with Adobo seasoning or salt and pepper.
8. Serve hot with steamed rice.

Asian Inspired

<u>"Chicken" Teriyaki</u>[36]

Serves 2 | Prep time: 10 min | Cook time: 10 min | Total 20 min

We love Japanese! This is the healthiest version of a family favorite.

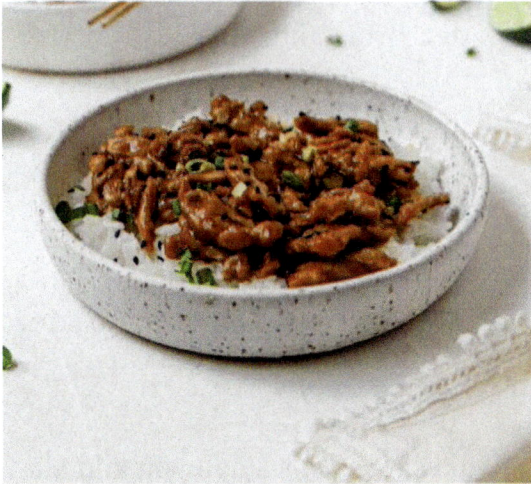

Ingredients:

Soy curl "chicken"

- o   3 cups water
- o   1 1/2 cups dry soy curls (<u>Amazon soy curls</u>) *may substitute GardeinChick'nstrips
- o   1/2 tablespoon sesame oil
- o   sliced medium sweet onion and bell pepper / chopped broccoli * to save time may use pre-sliced teriyaki vegetable prep kit

---

[36] Adapted from Mimi, M. (2021, September 18). *Vegan Teriyaki "Chicken" Soy Curls*. Daughter of Seitan. https://daughterofseitan.com/vegan-teriyaki-chicken-soy-curls/

Homemade teriyaki sauce (or 1/3 cup store bought)

- 1/4 cup reduced sodium soy sauce
- 1/3 cup vegetable broth (sub water)
- 3 tablespoons coconut sugar (sub brown sugar)
- 2 tablespoons rice vinegar
- 1/2 tablespoon sesame oil
- 1 teaspoon garlic powder
- 1/2 teaspoon ground ginger
- 1 tablespoon cornstarch + 2 tablespoons water (mixed together to form a slurry)
- Rice (white tastes better, brown healthier)
- Sesame seeds
- Lime wedges

Instructions:

1. For Gardein strips: stir fry in olive oil over medium heat about 5 mins. Otherwise, rehydrate the soy curls by adding to boiled water removed from heat, soaking for 8 minutes. They should be fully hydrated and tender. Drain and set aside.

2. For homemade teriyaki sauce. In a small pot, add all the ingredients for the teriyaki sauce except for the cornstarch. Bring to a rolling simmer over medium heat and simmer for 3 minutes, constantly stirring with a wooden spoon. Then mix in the cornstarch slurry, stir for 30 seconds, and remove from heat. The sauce should be thick and sticky, and will continue to thicken as it cools.

3. Cook the teriyaki soy curls in sesame oil over medium high heat. Lightly brown the soy curls (~5 minutes). Add vegetables and teriyaki sauce to coat the soy curls / strips and veggies.

4. Serve over rice topped with sesame seeds, or as desired. Leftovers will keep 5 days in the fridge.

Pad Thai with tofu[37]

Serves 4 | Prep time: 20 min | Cook time: 10 min | Total 30 min

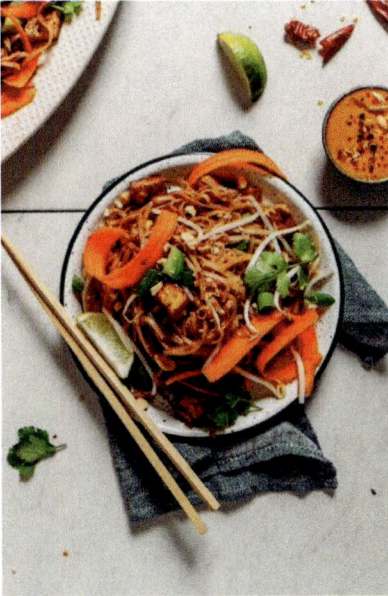

Ingredients:

Sauce

- o 1 ½ tsp tamarind paste / concentrate* (or sub additional 1 Tbsp / 15 ml lime juice as recipe is written)
- o 1/3 cup coconut aminos(or sub half the amount with tamari or soy sauce and work your way up as it's saltier)
- o 3 ½ Tbsp coconut sugar
- o 1 ½ tsp chili garlic sauce
- o 1 ½ Tbsp lime juice
- o 1-2 tsp Vegetarian Fish Sauce (or store-bought/ *optional*)

---

[37] Dana @ Minimalist Baker. (2022, October 11). *Easy Tofu Pad Thai*. Minimalist Baker. https://minimalistbaker.com/easy-tofu-pad-thai/

Stir Fry
- o 1 Tbsp sesame oil (if avoiding oil, omit and use a nonstick pan)
- o 1 cup cubed extra firm tofu
- o 2 Thai red chilies (fresh or dried), chopped OR 1/2 tsp chili flakes (*optional*)
- o 2 cloves garlic, minced (2 cloves yield ~1 Tbsp or 6 g)
- o 1 Tbsp coconut aminos(or tamari)
- o 1 cup bean sprouts
- o 1 cup chopped green onions
- o 1/3 cup chopped roasted salted peanuts

Noodles
- o 8 ounces Pad Thai rice noodles
- o Bean sprouts
- o Peanut sauce
- o Sriracha or Chili Garlic Sauce(we like Huy Fong Foods brand)

Instructions:

1. Heat tamarind, coconut aminos, coconut sugar, chili garlic sauce, lime juice, and optional vegetarian fish sauce over medium heat until barely simmering. Stir fry 30 sec and set aside.

2. Make sure that all of the ingredients for the stir-fry are prepared, including the cubed (shortly pressed) tofu, minced garlic, green onions, bean sprouts, and chopped peanuts. Prepare the optional peanut sauce now if you're serving it.

3. Place the Pad Thai noodles in a big bowl, then just add boiling water to cover them. Cook according to the directions on the box (often 5–6 minutes or until al dente). Stir and cover.

4. To prevent sticking, drain the noodles and mix with a little sesame oil. Place aside.

5. Over medium heat, preheat a big, rimmed skillet. Add the tofu and sauté for about 4 minutes, rotating it occasionally to ensure even browning. Garlic, coconut aminos (use caution as the coconut aminos can spatter), red pepper flakes or Thai chilies, and all of the above. Gently incorporate while tossing until just browned garlic is achieved.

6. Cook over medium-high heat, stirring occasionally (tongs are most helpful), for approximately 2-3 minutes or until the sauce has coated everything and the meal is hot.

7. Add noodles, Pad Thai sauce, bean sprouts, green onions, and peanuts.

8. To serve, plate the food with optional extras like cilantro, lime wedges, bean sprouts, peanut sauce, and sriracha or chile garlic sauce.

Chow Mein - Vegan[38]

Serves 4 | Prep time: 10 min | Cook time: 15 min | Total 25 min

Chinese food? Yes, please.

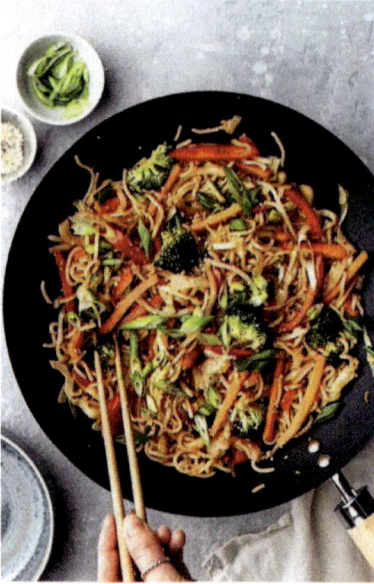

You Need:

Chow Mein Sauce
- 3 tbsp soy sauce
- 1 tbsp hoisin sauce
- 1 tbsp shaoxing wine or dry sherry
- 1.5 tsp sugar
- 1 tsp sesame oil
- 1 tsp sriracha (optional)

Stir Fry
- 3 garlic cloves, finely chopped
- 1 shallot, thinly sliced

---

[38] Tamsin, T. (2020, December 29). *Vegetable Chow Mein*. Cupful of Kale. https://cupfulofkale.com/vegan-vegetable-chow-mein/

- ○ 1 carrot, cut into thin strips
- ○ 1 red pepper, cut into thin strips
- ○ 1/2 white cabbage, shredded
- ○ 1/2 head broccoli, cut into small florets
- ○ 1.5 cups/150g bean sprouts
- ○ 300g chow mein noodles (or ramen)
- ○ 4 spring onions, chopped
- ○ Sesame seeds

Method:

1. Caramelize garlic and onion for about 20 seconds, tossing so they don't burn.
2. Add the broccoli and carrot and fry for 1-2 min.
3. Add the pepper, bean sprouts and cabbage and fry for 2 min. Toss well so they get cooked evenly.
4. Boil noodles, mix sauce ingredients
5. Add the chow mein sauce and noodles to the pan, stir well and serve!
6. Garnish with sesame seeds and serve.

Curry Cauliflower Soup[39]

Serves 8 | Prep time: 10 min | Cook time: 30 min | Total 40 min

Loaded with vegetables and seasoned with a winning flavor combination, this curried cauliflower soup is an exotic way to add more veggies into your family's diet!

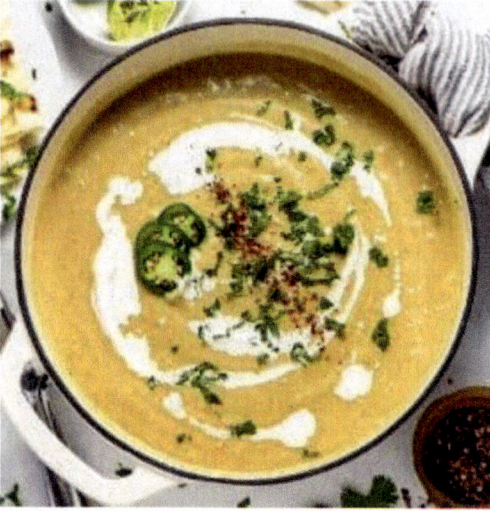

You Need:

- Pepper
- Salt
- Pinch cayenne
- Chili powder, .75 tbsp
- Curry powder, 1.5 tbsp
- Chopped head of cauliflower
- Vegetable broth, 3 c + 2 tbsp
- Diced garlic, two cloves
- Diced red onion, .5 c
- Diced red pepper, .5 c

---

[39] Adapted from Kylie. (2022, October 25). *Curried Cauliflower Soup [Vegan!]*. Midwest Foodie. https://midwestfoodieblog.com/curried-cauliflower-soup-vegan/

Method:

1. Add two tablespoons of broth and diced garlic to a pot and cook everything for a few minutes. Mix in the onion and peppers—Cook for a few more minutes.
2. Stir in the pepper, salt, cayenne, chili powder, curry powder, and cauliflower.
3. Add in the remaining broth and mix well.
4. Let this boil and then simmer for 25 minutes. Give the soup a little bit to cool, and then blend until smooth in a blender. Enjoy.

Sweet Potato, Spinach, and Lentil Dhal[40]

Serves 3 | Prep time: 15 min | Cook time: 30 min | Total 45 min

This is one of the most flavorful, fragrant, hearty soups I've ever experienced. After one bowl of this I feel full.

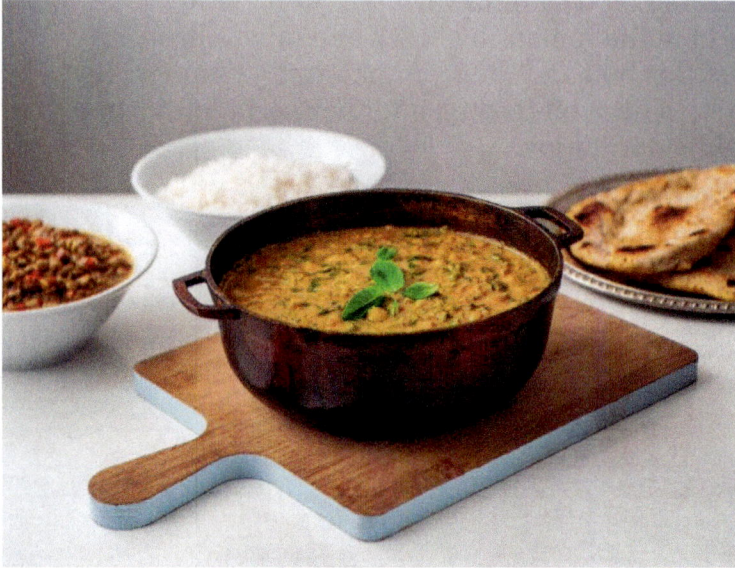

You Need:

- Sesame oil, 1 tbsp
- Crushed garlic clove
- Chopped red onion
- Sliced spring onions, 4 – sliced
- Spinach, .33 c
- Vegetable stock, 2.66 c
- Red split lentils, 1 c
- Sweet potatoes, 2
- Ground cumin, 1.5 tsp
- Ground turmeric, 1.5 tsp

---

[40] Adapted from Vegan, T. P. (2022, September 29). *Sweet Potato Dal with Lime (GF)*. The Pesky Vegan. https://thepeskyvegan.com/recipes/sweet-potato-dal/

- o Chopped red chili
- o Chopped ginger, small knob
- o Torn basil, ½ small pack

Method:

1. Caramelize onion in a large pot over medium heat.
2. Mix in the ginger, garlic, and red chili. Once fragrant, mix in the cumin and turmeric, cooking 1 minute.
3. Raise the heat and stir in the chopped sweet potatoes. Make sure that potatoes are well coated in the spices.
4. Stir in the stock and lentils. Sprinkle in some pepper and salt. Let this come up to a boil. Lower heat, cover and simmer for about 20 minutes. Make sure that the potatoes have become soft, along with the lentils.
5. Adjust seasoning to taste and add spinach. Once wilted, top with torn basil and chopped spring onions.

American Favorites

Award winning! Ultimate vegan chili[41]

Serves 4 | Prep time: 15 min | Cook time: 45 min | Total 60 min

The flavor of this chili is simply outstanding. I've never eaten chili faster than this!

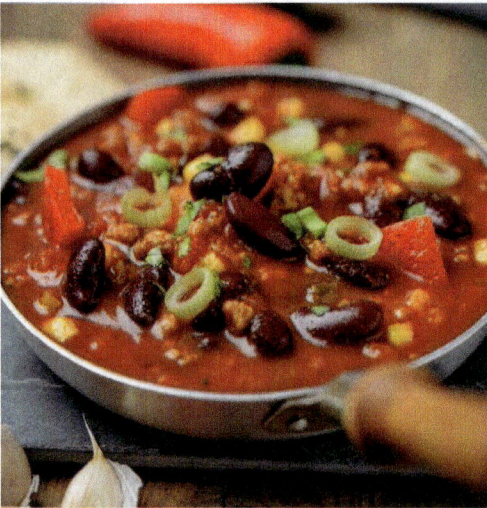

Ingredients

Meaty Tofu Crumbles
- o 2 tablespoons soy sauce *tamari for gluten free
- o 2 tablespoons nutritional yeast
- o 2 teaspoons chili powder
- o 1 teaspoon smoked paprika
- o (1) 14-ounce firm tofu

---

[41] Nora, N. (2022, November 14). *Ultimate Vegan Chili*. Nora Cooks. https://www.noracooks.com/ultimate-vegan-chili/

Chili

- o 2 tablespoons olive oil
- o 1 medium sweet onion, diced
- o 3-4 cloves garlic, minced
- o (2) 28-oz cans crushed tomatoes
- o (2) 15-oz cans black beans, drained and rinsed
- o (1) 15-oz can kidney beans, drained and rinsed
- o 1 cup water
- o 3 tablespoons chili powder
- o 2 teaspoons ground cumin
- o 1 tablespoon pure maple syrup
- o 1 tablespoon cocoa powder
- o 1 teaspoon smoked paprika
- o 1/4 teaspoon cayenne pepper
- o 1 teaspoon salt, or to taste

Instructions:

Prep Tofu Crumbles:

1. Place a parchment lined baking sheet in the oven and preheat it to 350 degrees.
2. Mix the soy sauce, nutritional yeast, chili powder, and smoked paprika in a large bowl into a paste. Using your hands, mash the tofu into the bowl, then stir it with a large spoon to thoroughly include it with the paste.
3. In the pan, distribute the tofu mixture evenly. Bake for 30 minutes with tofu being stirred halfway through. Start the chili once the tofu is in the oven.

While tofu bakes, make Chili:

1. Over medium heat, caramelize the chopped onion 3-4 minutes until translucent. Stir in the garlic and cook 1 minute
2. Add the rest of the chili ingredients, except the tofu, and stir to combine. Bring to a boil, then simmer for about 20 minutes

3. Stir in the tofu crumbles. Serve withtortilla chips, cilantro, tomatoes, hot sauce, vegan cheese shreds and chives, if desired

Notes:

- Replace tofu with vegan beef crumbles (Beyond Meat) if desired. Or simply add some of these instead: frozen corn, red bell peppers, sweet potatoes, carrots, or zucchini. Or add a cup of uncooked quinoa when you add the beans.
- Instant Pot version: Use the sauté feature and cook your onion and garlic, then add the rest of the ingredients except the tofu. Secure the lid and cook at high for 8 minutes. Stir in the tofu and serve.

Black Bean Burgers[42]

Live Long and Strong pizza[43]

2 medium pizzas (11 inch)
Prep time: 20 min | Cook time: 10 min | Total 30 min

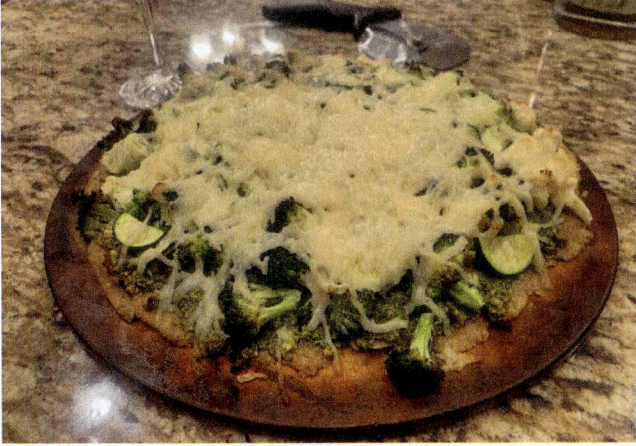

Ingredients:

- o 1 cup warm water, almost too hot for comfort (110 degrees)
- o 1 envelope rapid rise or instant yeast (2 1/4 teaspoons)
- o 1 tbsp sugar
- o 2 3/4 cup white whole wheat flour
- o 1/4 cup nutritional yeast
- o 1 tsp salt
- o Pesto sauce, e.g. Trader Joe's vegan pesto
- o Dairy free cheese, e.g.Daiya mozzarella
- o 1 cup of chopped broccoli and cauliflower florets

---

[42] Based on *Homemade Black Bean Veggie Burgers*. (2022, June 14). Allrecipes. https://www.allrecipes.com/recipe/85452/homemade-black-bean-veggie-burgers/

[43] Adapted from Nora, N. (2021, August 9). *Easiest Whole Wheat Oil Free Pizza*. Nora Cooks. https://www.noracooks.com/easiest-whole-wheat-oil-free-pizza/

Instructions:

1. Preheat oven to 425°F.
2. Whisk the warm water, yeast and sugar in a large bowl, or your standing mixer bowl. Allow it to sit for 5 minutes.
3. Add the flour, nutritional yeast and salt. If kneading mix everything together with a wooden spoon until combined, then knead on a lightly floured surface for about 5 minutes until you have a smooth ball of dough (use the dough hook on setting 2 for 5 minutes if using standing mixer).
4. Halve the dough. On a lightly floured countertop, roll out to about an 11-inch diameter. You should get two good sized pizzas.
5. Transfer to non-stick baking pans.
6. Add your pesto sauce, veggies and vegan cheese. Bake for 8 minutes for a soft crust or 10 minutes for a crispy crust.

NOTES: The broccoli and cauliflower will release sulforaphane when chewed, which has been shown to be heart healthy and anti-cancer (see Chapter 2 in Book 1). You could eat broccoli sprouts or brussels sprouts once a day if you want the highest concentration for these health benefits.

Desserts - yes you can make desserts without dairy!

Banana Energy Cookies[44]

3 dozen |Prep time: 20 min | Cook time: 20 minutes | Total 40 min

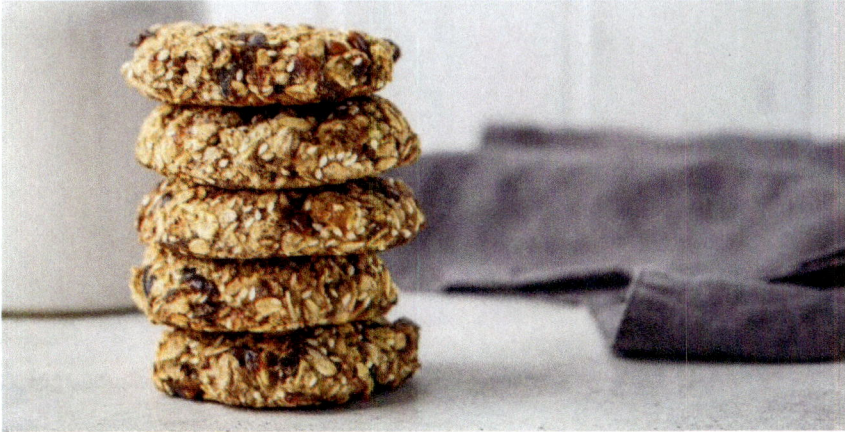

Kid-tested and mother-approved!

You Need:

- ○ Vanilla, 1 tsp
- ○ Vegetable oil, .33 c
- ○ Chopped dates, 1 c
- ○ Rolled oats, 2 c
- ○ Bananas, 3

Method:

1. Preheat the oven to 350 degrees.

---

44 Adapted from Veganista, S. T. J. |. (2022, February 16). *3 INGREDIENT BANANA OATMEAL COOKIES*. THE SIMPLE VEGANISTA. https://simple-veganista.com/chocolate-chip-banana-bread-bites/

2. Mash up the bananas and then mix in the remaining ingredients, making sure that you mix everything well. Let this sit for 15 minutes to thicken. Drop teaspoon-sized drops of the dough onto an ungreased baking sheet.
3. Bake for 20 minutes or until browned.

Dairy-Free Pineapple Whip[45]

Serves 3 | Prep time: 10 min

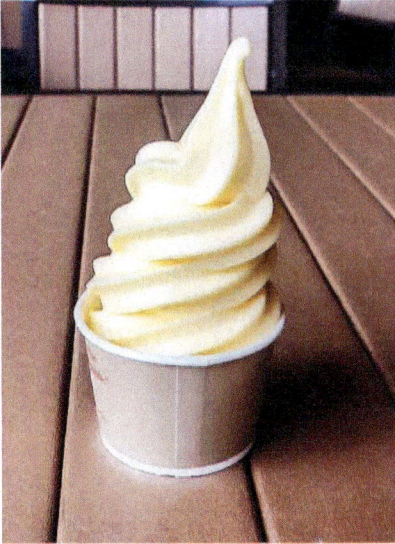

A homemade version of the famous Dole Whip found at Disney World! Taste the magic!

You Need:

- o 1 pound frozen pineapple
- o 1 can full fat coconut milk, chilled for 24 hours (use only solid white coconut cream in this recipe)
- o 1 tablespoon pure maple syrup

Method:

1. Blend all the ingredients at high speed. Put the top on and insert the tamper through the lid's opening. Use the tamper to continuously push the frozen pineapple down into the blade of the blender while it is running

---

45 Gordon, E. (2022, June 24). *Easy Dairy-Free Dole Whip (Pineapple Soft Serve)*. Eating by Elaine. https://www.eatingbyelaine.com/dole-whip-aka-vegan-pineapple-soft-serve/

at medium speed until the mixture is creamy smooth. This could take one or two minutes. Serve as is.

2. For the soft-serve swirl: pour the Dole Whip from the blender into a sizable plastic bag and seal. Then, make a little slit in one of the bag's lower corners. Use a swirling motion to squeeze the bag into your serving bowls or cups. Enjoy right away!

Peanut butter cookies[46]

2 dozen | Prep time: 10 mins | Cook time: 12 mins | Total 22 mins

Soft, chewy, peanut butter goodness.

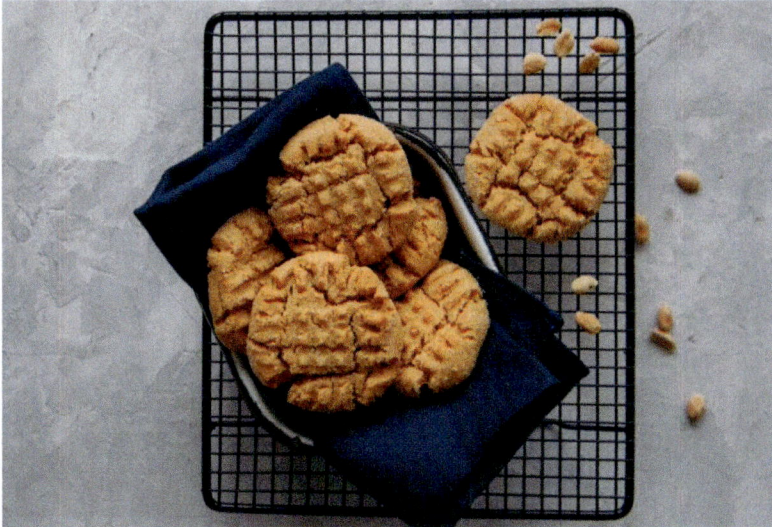

Ingredients:

- o 1/2 cup vegan butter, softened
- o 3/4 cup creamy peanut butter
- o 1/2 cup granulated sugar
- o 1/2 cup brown sugar
- o 2 tablespoons almond milk
- o 1 teaspoon vanilla
- o 1 1/4 cups all purpose flour
- o 3/4 teaspoon baking soda
- o 1/2 teaspoon baking powder
- o 2 tablespoons cornstarch
- o 1/4 teaspoon salt

---

[46] Nora, N. (2021, August 4). *Vegan Peanut Butter Cookies (1 Bowl)*. Nora Cookshttps://www.noracooks.com/vegan-peanut-butter-cookies/

- 1/4 cup granulated sugar, optional for rolling

Instructions:

1. Preheat the oven to 350°F and cover a baking sheet with parchment paper. For rolling the cookies in, add 1/4 cup sugar to a small bowl and set it aside.
2. Mix the vegan butter, peanut butter, and sugars in a large bowl. Add the almond milk and vanilla, combining thoroughly. A hand mixer, stand mixer, or a big wooden spoon can be used.
3. Add the flour, then add the salt, baking soda, baking powder, cornstarch, and baking powder. Until a dough is formed, stir (or use a mixer). It will be a heavy, sticky dough.
4. Roll balls of dough and press the tops of each one to create a crisscross pattern as you place them on the prepared baking sheet.
5. The cookies will seem a little underdone and mushy, but they continue to set as they cool. Bake the cookies for 10 to 12 minutes, or until they are very faintly golden brown.
6. Prior to transferring to a wire rack, let the items cool on the baking sheet for about 5 minutes. For about a week, these cookies will be OK at room temperature.

Notes:

1. Makes 20-24 cookies.
2. May sub coconut oil, softened, for the vegan butter. For crunchy peanut butter cookies, simply bake 2-3 minutes longer. I prefer them soft, but I know some people like crunchy.
3. **To store:** will keep for up to 5 days covered at room temperature.

Chapter 3

Ten Days to Transform Your Health: The 10 Day Eat Real Food Plan

"For the vast majority of chronic diseases, it's the same lifestyle recommendations because they really are the same disease... essentially a whole food, plant-based diet."

- Dr. Ornish, bestselling author of Undo It! How Simple Lifestyle Changes Can Reverse Most Chronic Diseases

By now you may have decided to try a ten day diet change, whether it be for your health and longevity, the environment, peak performance, or maybe because now it looks easy and delicious! Below is your 10 Day Eat Real Food Plan. You will see breakfast is optional but it may be easier initially to skip it for a day or two, then have it, etc.

These meals are tasty, healthy, affordable and most serve four people in 30-45 minutes. If you have leftovers they will keep a few days in the fridge and you won't have to cook as often! My mom, a former chef, requested several of these recipes including the Savory sausage pasta and Creamy risotto...

The 10 Day Eat Real Food Plan: ten days of savory 30 minute meals, whole foods plant-based

Day	Breakfast (optional)	Lunch 30min meals*	Dinner 30-45min meals**
1	Skip it	Mexican bean salad	Savory sausage pasta
2	Smoothie e.g. peanut dream smoothie	Chipotle bean burrito dairy free or Black bean burritos	Chef Special! Mom's herb crusted meatloaf
3	Blueberry smoothie bowl	Garden salad with walnuts or mixed nuts	Vegan haluski: Polish comfort food
4	Skip it	"Chicken" Teriyaki	Award winning! Ultimate vegan chili
5	Skip it	Ancient grains bowl (True Foods recipe)	Spaghetti and Beyond Meatballs
6	Berry walnut oatmeal	Black bean and avocado bowl	Black bean burgers
7	Breakfast of tofu champions	Quinoa Gado-Gado bowl	Brown rice stir fry with caramelized onion and broccoli
8	Skip it	Arugula quinoa bowl	Live Long and Strong Pizza or Garden pizza
9	Skip it	Pad thai with tofu	Creamy mushroom risotto

| 10 | 2 bananas | Vegan Chow Mein | Cuban black bean soup |

* If you have more time to cook, you may want to look up more involved recipes, e.g.noracooks.com
** You can add an appetizer like vegan garlic toast if desired. You may also want to add a side of steamed brussels sprouts or broccoli sprouts every day (cruciferous vegetables)... and remember to use whole grains.

If you don't want to cook one day or want a quick meal these are always on standby: salad with nuts, corn chips and salsa, garlic hummus with raw vegetables and pita chips, whole grain toast with natural peanut butter, or Trader Joe's roasted potatoes with peppers and onion tossed with corn.

Breakfast

Please note you're encouraged to either skip breakfast or eat only fruit before noon. Keep in mind humans did not evolve eating three meals a day. In fact, no animals regularly eat anytime they want; there is rarely an abundant food source in the wild. Many eat once a day at a maximum. While we are fortunate to have abundant food, it does not mean we have to eat three times a day.

If you eat all your food at lunch and dinner you will reap health and longevity benefits from intermittent fasting (see Dr. Longo's research on time-restricted feeding outlined in *Life Force* Chapter 12)[47]. For example, when fasting the blood glucose levels drop and cause a decrease in the production of insulin. When this happens, the body sends out a signal to start burning fat for energy.

Intermittent fasting is a lifestyle and dietary choice, but those who end up being the most successful are those who

---

[47] Robbins, Tony et al. (2022). *Life Force: How New Breakthroughs in Precision Medicine Can Transform the Quality of Your Life & Those You Love.* Simon & Schuster. pg 286-291

accept it as a lifestyle almost immediately. Once you decide to do it, it's pretty easy after the first couple of days. The main point is to eat less food and eat less often.

If you would like to have something before noon please see the smoothie section in Chapter 2. You might also consider eating only fruit before noon until morning food cravings subside. Now that you've decided to eat whole foods plant-based for ten days, you may want to refer to the recipes from the previous chapter (featuring food photos). For readers who prefer it faster, here are the recipes in order of the 10 day eat real food plan.

Lunch recipes

Day 1: Mexican bean salad

Serves 4 | Prep time 15min | Total time 45min

Ingredients

- 1 (15 ounce) can black beans, rinsed and drained
- 1 (15 ounce) can red kidney beans, rinsed and drained
- 1 (15 ounce) can cannellini beans, rinsed and drained
- 1 green bell pepper, chopped
- 1 red bell pepper, chopped
- 1 (10 ounce) package frozen corn kernels, thawed
- 1 red onion, diced
- ½ cup olive oil
- ½ cup red wine vinegar
- ¼ cup chopped fresh cilantro
- 2 tablespoons fresh lime juice
- 1 tablespoon lemon juice
- 1 clove garlic, crushed
- 2 tablespoons white sugar
- 1 tablespoon salt
- 1 ½ teaspoons ground cumin

- 1 ½ teaspoons ground black pepper
- ½ teaspoon chili powder, or to taste
- 1 dash hot pepper sauce, or to taste

Directions

1. Combine beans, bell peppers, corn, and red onion in a large bowl.
2. Whisk olive oil, vinegar, cilantro, lime juice, lemon juice, garlic, sugar, salt, cumin, and black pepper together in a small bowl. Season with chili powder and hot sauce.
3. Pour dressing over bean mixture and toss well. Refrigerate until chilled, 30min (until corn is thawed). Serve cold.

Day 2: Black Bean Burritos

"Serves 6   Prep time: 10 min   Cook time: 15 min   Total 25 min"

You Need:

For the Red Rice:
- Dry white rice, 1 c
- Water, .25 c
- Diced fresh tomato, 1 c
- Vegetable broth, 1 c
- Minced garlic, two cloves
- Diced white onion, 1 medium – reserve .25 cup
- Olive oil, 1 tbsp

For the Chili Lime Black Beans:
- Black beans, two cans – drained and rinsed
- Cumin, 2 tsp
- Chili powder, .75 tsp
- Pepper, 1 tsp
- Sea salt, 1 tsp
- Minced garlic, one clove

- o Lime juice, 2 tbsp

For Burritos:
- o Cilantro, .25 c per burrito
- o Guacamole, .25 c per burrito
- o Grated carrot, .25 c per burrito
- o Large wheat or corn tortillas

Method:

1. Cook the garlic and onion on some of the oil for about six to seven minutes until fragrant.
2. Add in the tomato, water, broth, and rice and cook, covered, until the rice is cooked through. This takes about 10 to 15 minutes.
3. Add in the reserved onion and garlic with the beans, pepper, chili powder, salt, cumin, and lime juice. With a potato masher, mash up some of the beans and cook for five to eight minutes until heated.
4. When the beans and rice are done, add to a large tortilla with your favorite toppings.

Day 3: Garden Salad

For lunch, enjoy a quick power greens salad topped with mixed nuts including walnuts and pecans. Dress with Italian vinaigrette of choice.

Day 4: "Chicken" Teriyaki

Serves 2 | Prep Time 10 min | Cook 40 min | Total 50 min

Ingredients:

Soy curl "chicken"

- 3 cups water
- 1 1/2 cups dry soy curls ([Amazon soy curls](#)) *may substitute GardeinChick'nstrips
- 1/2 tablespoon sesame oil
- sliced medium sweet onion and bell pepper / chopped broccoli * to save time may use pre-sliced teriyaki vegetable prep kit

Homemade teriyaki sauce (or 1/3 cup store bought)

- 1/4 cup reduced sodium soy sauce
- 1/3 cup vegetable broth (sub water)
- 3 tablespoons coconut sugar (sub brown sugar)
- 2 tablespoons rice vinegar
- 1/2 tablespoon sesame oil
- 1 teaspoon garlic powder
- 1/2 teaspoon ground ginger
- 1 tablespoon cornstarch + 2 tablespoons water (mixed together to form a slurry)
- Rice (white tastes better, brown healthier)
- Sesame seeds
- Lime wedges

Instructions:

1. For Gardein strips: stir fry in olive oil over medium heat about 5 mins. Otherwise, rehydrate the soy curls by adding to boiled water removed from heat, soaking for 8 minutes. They should be fully hydrated and tender. Drain and set aside.
2. For homemade teriyaki sauce. In a small pot, add all the ingredients for the teriyaki sauce except for the cornstarch. Bring to a rolling simmer over medium heat and simmer for 3 minutes, constantly stirring with a wooden spoon. Then mix in the cornstarch slurry, stir for 30 seconds, and remove from heat. The sauce should be thick and sticky, and will continue to thicken as it cools.
3. Cook the teriyaki soy curls in sesame oil over medium high heat. Lightly brown the soy curls (~5 minutes).

Add vegetables and teriyaki sauce to coat the soy curls / strips and veggies.

4. Serve over rice topped with sesame seeds, or as desired. Leftovers will keep 5 days in the fridge.

Day 5: Ancient Grains Bowl (from True Food Kitchen)

Prep Time 10 min | Cook 40 min | Total 50 min

Ingredients

- 2 sweet potatoes, peeled and diced 1/2"
- 1 small red onion, peeled and sliced
- 1-2 tablespoons extra virgin olive oil
- sea salt and pepper to taste
- 2 servings ancient grains of your choice, cooked to package instructions, e.g. barley, millet, sorghum. You can also use multicolor quinoa (cooks in 15min)
- 1 1/2 tablespoons honey
- 1 tablespoon Sambal Oelek (add more or less depending on how you like the heat!)
- 1 tablespoon dijon mustard
- 1/2 cup snow peas
- ¾ cup mushrooms, sliced
- 1 ripe avocado, sliced
- 1 tablespoon chives for garnish
- Optional: pesto sauce (If you don't want to make your own, you could buy at Trader Joe's)

Method:

1. Preheat oven to 425°F, line rimmed cookie sheet with parchment paper, set aside
2. Add potatoes and onion, drizzle with olive oil, sprinkle with sea salt and freshly ground pepper, toss.
3. Bake in oven 35 minutes
4. Cook grains ~20-40min depending on grains on hand.
5. While grains cook, slice chives and mushrooms. Whisk together honey, sambal oelek, and dijon mustard, set aside
6. When potatoes are almost done (crispy browned) add mushrooms and snow peas to the pan and set timer for 5 more minutes.

7. Divide cooked grains into two bowls, top with veggies, drizzle with sauce from step 5, leaving some in a small bowl to use as needed. Add avocado, chives. Add pesto if using. Enjoy!

Day 6: Black Bean and Avocado Bowl

"Serves 1 Prep time: 10 min Cook time: 10 min Total 20 min"

You Need:

- Pepper
- Cilantro leaves, 2 tbsp
- Salt
- Black beans, warmed, .5 c
- Olive oil, 1 tsp
- Thinly sliced medium radish, 1
- Grape tomatoes, .5 c
- Thinly slice avocado, .5
- Corn kernels from one ear

Method:

1. Add the beans into a shallow bowl and set to the side. Place a small skillet on medium heat. Add olive oil and allow to warm up. Place tomatoes into skillet and cook until charred. Shake the pan to turn the tomatoes. Put the tomatoes beside the beans in a bowl.
2. Add corn to the skillet and heat through. Put the corn beside the tomatoes. Add cilantro, sliced radish, and sliced avocado to the bowl. Sprinkle on pepper and salt. Enjoy.

Day 7: Quinoa Gado-Gado Bowl

"Serves 2 Prep time: 10 min Cook time: 20 minutes Total 30 min"

You Need:

For Spicy Peanut Sauce:
- Water, 3 – 4 tbsp
- Creamy peanut butter, .33 c
- Chili garlic sauce, 1 tsp
- Soy sauce, 1 tbsp
- Lime juice, 3 tbsp
- Maple syrup, 2 – 3 tbsp

For Gado-Gado:
- Thinly sliced carrots, 2
- Quinoa, .5 c
- Thinly shredded red cabbage, .66 c
- Water, 1 c
- Mung bean sprouts, .75 c
- Trimmed green beans, 1 c
- Thinly sliced red bell pepper, .5

Method:
1. Cook quinoa according to the directions on the package.
2. Steam the green beans while the quinoa is cooking. Once they are steamed, add them to ice water to stop them from cooking. Set to the side.
3. To make the peanut sauce: add the chili garlic sauce, peanut butter, maple syrup, lime juice, and soy sauce to a bowl and mix everything together. Add one tablespoon at a time until it makes a pourable sauce. You do not want this too thin.
4. Taste and adjust seasonings if needed.
5. To serve equally, divide quinoa into two bowls. Top with carrots, mung bean sprouts, red bell pepper, and green beans. Drizzle over the peanut sauce. Can

garnish with a sprinkle of red pepper flakes, lime wedges, or cilantro, if desired.

Day 8: Arugula Quinoa Bowl

"Serves 1 Prep time: 10 min Cook time: 15 minutes Total 15 min"

Ingredients:

- o Pepper
- o Salt
- o Crumbled vegan cheese, 2 tsp, e.g. vegan parmesan
- o Sherry vinegar, 1 tbsp
- o Chopped walnuts, 2 tbsp
- o Olive oil, 2 tsp
- o Chopped peaches, .25 c (optional - better to eat 10 min before rest of salad)
- o Arugula, 1 c
- o Sliced avocado, .5
- o Cooked quinoa, .75 c
- o lemon vinaigrette dressing

Method:
1. Put quinoa in boiling water, reduce heat and simmer 15min until water absorbed
2. Whisk together pepper, salt, oil, and vinegar in a small bowl.
3. Put the arugula into the bottom of a medium bowl. Place the walnuts, peaches, avocados, and quinoa around the sides of the bowl. Drizzle dressing over and sprinkle on cheese.

Day 9: Pad Thai with tofu

Serves 4 | Prep time 20 min | Cook 10 min | Total 30 min

Ingredients:

SAUCE
- o 1 ½ tsp tamarind paste (or sub additional 1 Tbsp / 15 ml lime juice as recipe is written)
- o 1/3 cup coconut aminos (or sub half the amount with tamari or soy sauce and work your way up as it's saltier)
- o 3 ½ Tbsp coconut sugar
- o 1 ½ tsp chili garlic sauce
- o 1 ½ Tbsp lime juice
- o 1-2 tsp vegetarian fish sauce (or store-bought // *optional*)

STIR FRY
- o 1 Tbsp sesame oil (if avoiding oil, omit and use a nonstick pan)
- o 1 cup cubed extra firm tofu
- o 2 Thai red chilies (fresh or dried), chopped OR 1/2 tsp chili flakes (*optional*)
- o 2 cloves garlic, minced (2 cloves yield ~1 Tbsp or 6 g)
- o 1 Tbsp coconut aminos(or tamari)
- o 1 cup bean sprouts
- o 1 cup chopped green onions
- o 1/3 cup chopped roasted salted peanuts

NOODLES
- o 8 ouncespad thai rice noodles(We like Annie Chun's brand)
- o Bean sprouts
- o Peanut sauce
- o Sriracha or chili garlic sauce(we like Huy Fong Foods brand)

Instructions:

1. Heat tamarind, coconut aminos, coconut sugar, chili garlic sauce, lime juice, and optional vegetarian fish sauce over medium heat until barely simmering. Stir fry 30 sec and set aside.
2. Make sure that all of the ingredients for the stir-fry are prepared, including the cubed (shortly pressed) tofu, minced garlic, green onions, bean sprouts, and chopped peanuts. Prepare the optional peanut sauce now if you're serving it.
3. Place the Pad Thai noodles in a big bowl, then just add boiling water to cover them. Cook according to the directions on the box (often 5–6 minutes or until al dente). Stir and cover.
4. To prevent sticking, drain the noodles and mix with a little sesame oil. Place aside.
5. Over medium heat, preheat a big, rimmed skillet. Add the tofu and sauté for about 4 minutes, rotating it occasionally to ensure even browning. Garlic, coconut aminos (use caution as the coconut aminos can spatter), red pepper flakes or Thai chilies, and all of the above. Gently incorporate while tossing until just browned garlic is achieved.
6. Cook over medium-high heat, stirring occasionally (tongs are most helpful), for approximately 2-3 minutes or until the sauce has coated everything and the meal is hot.
7. Add noodles, Pad Thai sauce, bean sprouts, green onions, and peanuts.
8. To serve, plate the food with optional extras like cilantro, lime wedges, bean sprouts, peanut sauce, and sriracha or chile garlic sauce.

Day 10: Chow Mein

"Serves 4 Prep time: 10 min Cook time: 15 min Total 25 min"

You Need:

- o   Shredded cabbage, 2 c
- o   Sliced celery, 3 stalks
- o   Diced onion
- o   Olive oil, 2 tbsp
- o   Yaki Soba, 2 packages – seasoning packets discarded
- o   Pepper, .25 tsp
- o   Grated ginger, 2 tsp
- o   Brown sugar, 1 tbsp
- o   Minced garlic, 3 cloves
- o   Reduced sodium soy sauce, .25 c

Method:

1. Start by mixing together the pepper, ginger, brown sugar, garlic, and soy sauce.
2. Add the Yaki Soba to boiling water. Cook for one to two minutes and drain.
3. Pour in some oil and then toss in the celery and onion. Let this cook for three to four minutes or until they become tender. Mix in the cabbage and cook for another minute.
4. Mix in the noodles and the soy sauce mixture—Cook for two minutes.
5. Enjoy.

Dinner Recipes

Day 1: Savory sausage pasta

Serves 2 | Total time 30 min

A former chef requested this recipe. Enjoy!

Ingredients:

- ½ Spanish or vidalia onion
- 1 tsp Minced garlic (1 clove)
- 1 lb ground plant sausage e.g. Impossible sausage savory
- Extra virgin olive oil, cold pressed (EVOO), enough to thinly coat pan
- ½ lb whole grain fusilli or penne pasta
- ½ tsp vegetable Better than Bouillon in 1 cup water / 1 can vegetable broth*
- Paprika and ground pepper

* The bouillon in water is much cheaper with less waste than buying pre-packed vegetable broth. It also tastes better.

Directions:

1. Brown sausage in EVOO, sprinkle with dash of paprika, dice onion, boil pasta
2. Drain sausage on paper towel, dump oil (may skip this step)
3. Add fresh EVOO, teaspoon minced garlic (1 clove)
4. Caramelize diced onion
5. Add sausage and vegetable broth
6. Reduce heat from boil to simmer, add ground pepper if you want more bite

Day 2: Chef special! Mom's herb-crusted meatloaf

Serves 3 | 15min prep | 30min cook time | 45min total

Ingredients:

- o 1 lb Beyond Meat plant-based ground
- o 1 tsp minced garlic (1 clove in garlic press)
- o 1/2 vidalia onion diced
- o 5 tbsp Marinara sauce
- o 1 tbsp each of sage, basil, rosemary
- o 1 cup brown precooked rice
- o 2 tbsp sea salt
- o 2 tbsp olive or canola oil
- o Optional: a few small potatoes and carrots cut up in quarters with the same spices; arrange on foil around the loaf, then drizzle olive oil lightly on potatoes and carrots only . Note potatoes and carrots have to be pre boiled and cooled but only boiled for 5 minutes as otherwise not cooked.

Directions:

1. Pre-heat oven to 400F, boil pot of water
2. Sauté onion and garlic in olive oil until golden, drain off most of the oil but leave a little
3. While caramelizing onion, in a medium mixing bowl use a wooden spatula to poke holes into plant ground. Mix in herbs and marinara
4. Add drained onions and garlic, mix all together.
5. Once blended form into loaf or football shape on foil lined pan
6. Then add a little marinara over top of the loaf, tent with foil but be sure it doesn't stick to the loaf. So it's tight around the edges but elevated on the top.
7. Bake 30min
8. Add rice to pot, stir in 1 tsp vegetable Bouillon, and simmer on medium until water absorbed, ~15min

9. Plate strips of loaf on a bed of rice, season to taste with sea salt. May also season rice with Italian herb grinder

Day 3: Vegan haluski - polish comfort food

Serves 3 | Prep time: 15 mins | Cooking time: 30 mins

Ingredients:

- o 2 Tbsp canola oil or vegan butter or olive oil
- o 1 large sweet onion
- o 6 cups shredded cabbage (about 1 small head, red or green)
- o 1/2 tsp garlic powder
- o 1/4 tsp turmeric (optional)
- o sea salt to taste, fresh ground pepper to taste
- o 1 block firm tofu (1lb/450g) (optional, will serve 2 without it)
- o 16oz rice noodles (international aisle with thai food packets)
- o 1/4 cup vegan butter, e.g. Earth Balance

Method:

1. Boil the noodles according to package directions, drain and rinse.
2. Slice onion in long thin slices.
3. Put oil in the bottom of a large pot and add the onion, sprinkle with a little salt, and cook on low heat for about 8 minutes
4. Cut the cabbage into long skinny pieces about 1/8 of an inch wide, while the onions are cooking.
5. Add the cabbage, sprinkle with salt and pepper, and turn up the heat to medium.
6. Add tofu if desired — drain, press and crumble the tofu block into the pot.

7. Add the garlic powder, turmeric, salt, and pepper and let it all cook for about 10 minutes stirring frequently until cabbage wilts down and loses its bright color.
8. Rinse the noodles again to make them wet and avoid sticking to each other.
9. Add the noodles and butter to the pot and mix well and cook for another minute or two until all the butter has melted and is coating the noodles and veggies.
10. Turn off the heat and add additional salt and fresh ground pepper to taste.

Day 4: Award winning! Ultimate vegan chili

Serves 4 | Prep 15min | Cook 45min | Total time 60min

Ingredients:

Meaty Tofu Crumbles:

- Firm tofu, 14 oz
- Smoked paprika, 1 tsp
- Chili powder, 2 tsp
- Nutritional yeast, 2 tbsp
- Soy sauce, 2 tbsp – tamari for gluten free

Chili:

- Salt, 1 tsp
- Cayenne pepper, .25 tsp
- Smoked paprika, 1 tsp
- Cocoa powder, 1 tbsp
- Pure maple syrup, 1 tbsp
- Ground cumin, 2 tsp
- Chili powder, 3 tbsp
- Water, 1 c
- Kidney beans, 15 oz – drained and rinsed
- Black beans, 2 15 oz cans – drained and rinsed

- Crushed tomatoes, 2 28 oz cans
- Minced garlic, 3 to 4 cloves
- Diced onion
- Olive oil, 2 tbsp

Instructions:

For the Tofu Crumbles:

1. Preheat the oven to 350 degrees F and line abaking sheet withparchment paper.
2. In a large bowl, mix together the soy sauce, nutritional yeast, chili powder and smoked paprika. It will be pasty. Now crumble the tofu into the bowl with your hands, and mix together using a large spoon until well combined with the paste.
3. Spread the tofu mixture evenly in the pan. Place in the oven and bake for 30 minutes, stirring the tofu halfway through. Once the tofu is in the oven, start the chili.

While tofu bakes make Chili:

1. In a larger pot over medium heat, add the olive oil. Add the chopped onion and sauté 3-4 minutes until translucent. Add in the garlic and cook for 1 more minute, stirring constantly.
2. Now add all the rest of the chili ingredients, except the tofu, and stir to combine. Bring to a boil, then lower the heat and simmer for about 20 minutes, until the tofu crumbles are done baking.
3. If a thicker consistency is desired, use an immersion blender and blend just a few times. Do this before you add the tofu.
4. Once the tofu crumbles are done, stir them into the pot. All done! Serve withcornbread, tortilla chips, cilantro, tomatoes, hot sauce, vegan cheese shreds and chives, if desired.

Notes:

- May omit the tofu crumbles if desired, or replace them with vegan beef crumbles (Beyond Meat). Or simply add some vegetables instead, like frozen corn, red bell peppers, sweet potatoes, carrots or zucchini. Or add a cup of uncooked quinoa when you add the beans.
- Instant Pot version: Use the sauté feature and cook your onion and garlic, then add the rest of the ingredients (except the tofu, bake that in the oven like normal). Secure the lid and cook at high pressure for 8 minutes. Stir in the tofu crumbles and serve.

Day 5: Spaghetti with Beyond Meatballs

Serves 4 | Prep time: 20 min | Cook time: 35 min | Total 55 min

You Need:

- Dried parsley, 1.5 tsp
- Vegan breadcrumbs, 1 tbsp
- Beyond Meat Ground, 1 lb.
- Pepper, .5 tsp - divided
- Salt, 1.25 tsp – divided
- Oregano, 1 tsp
- Tomato sauce, 8 oz
- Minced garlic, three cloves
- Chopped medium onion
- Olive oil, 4 tbsp – divide
- Whole peeled tomatoes, 28 oz can – drained, juice reserved
- Spaghetti, 12 oz
- Onion powder, .25 tsp
- Garlic powder, .25 tsp

Method:

1. Dice the tomatoes and place them back with the juices.
2. Add two tablespoons of the oil to a pot with the garlic and onion. Cook for about two minutes, stirring. Add in the tomatoes and their juice, a quarter teaspoon of pepper, half a teaspoon of salt, oregano, and tomato sauce. Let this come up to a simmer, and let it cook as you fix the meatballs.
3. Combine the beef substitute with the onion powder, garlic powder, remaining pepper, remaining salt, parsley, and breadcrumbs. Once mixed together, roll them into one-and-a-half-inch balls.
4. Add slightly salted water to a pot and let it boil. Add in the spaghetti, cooking for 12 minutes.
5. Meanwhile, add the rest of the oil to a skillet and cook the meatballs. Turn them occasionally, cooking for about ten minutes.
6. Pour the sauce over the meatballs and mix. Simmer for an additional ten minutes.
7. Serve spaghetti topped with sauce and meatballs.

Day 6: Black Bean Burgers

Serves 4 | Prep time: 10 min | Cook time: 20 min | Total 30 min

You Need:

- Hot sauce, 1 tsp
- Cumin, 1 tbsp
- 1 Vegan Egg, e.g. Just Egg
- Peeled Garlic, three cloves
- ½ red onion sliced into wedges
- Chili powder, 1 tbsp
- ½ of a chopped green bell pepper
- Rinsed black beans, 16 oz can
- Whole grain bun (with sesame seeds)

Method:

1. First, you will need to decide if you are going to bake the burgers or grill them. If you are baking them, have your oven heated to 375. If you are grilling them, preheat your grill to high.
2. Mash the beans up in a bowl until it comes together to create a thick paste.
3. Add the vegetables to a processor and let everything chop finely. Mix this into the mashed beans.
4. Mix in the hot sauce, cumin, chili powder, and "egg" until it all makes a thick mixture. When you ball some up in your hand and squeeze it together, it should hold its shape. Divide the bean mixture into fourths and shape them into burgers.
5. Lay the burgers out on the grill and let them grill for eight minutes on each side. If baking, place them on a cookie sheet and then let them cook for about ten minutes.
6. Make your burger the way you like and enjoy.

Day 7: Brown Rice Stir Fry

Serves 4 | Prep time: 10 min | Cook time: 25 min | Total 35 min

You Need:

- Brown rice, 1.5 c pre-boiled
- Pepper and salt
- Ground cumin, .5 tsp
- Broccoli florets from 2 small heads
- One thinly sliced bell pepper
- Thinly sliced onion, 3 small
- Minced garlic, 1 tsp (1 crushed clove)
- Canola oil or olive oil, 2 tbsp
- Soy sauce to taste

Method:

1. Bring rice to a boil then simmer for 20 min on medium heat.
2. While rice cooks, caramelize the onions in 1-2 tbsp oil.
3. Lower the heat, add peppers, stirring often, until caramelized ~10min. Add garlic. May add soy sauce here if teriyaki flavor is desired.
4. Remove half of the onions to the rice pot. Continue to cook the other half as the rice is cooking.
5. Add the rest of the oil to a small pot. Add the cumin and the broccoli with a touch of water. Cover, and let the broccoli steam for 4-5 minutes. Stir this into the cooked rice. Garnish with the reserved onions and serve with soy sauce.

Day 8: Garden Pizza

Serves 4 |Prep time: 10 min | Cook time: 30 minutes | Total 40 min

You Need:

- Pepper
- Salt
- Torn basil, .25 c
- Whole wheat pizza dough, 12 oz
- Lemon zest, .5 tsp
- Water, 8 c
- Lemon juice, 1 tsp
- Asparagus spears, trimmed and sliced diagonally in half, one bunch
- Small zucchini turned into "noodles."
- Snap peas, 1 c
- Shredded vegan cheese, 3 oz
- Cashew ricotta cheese, .66 c
- Minced garlic, one clove
- Coconut milk, 2 tbsp

Method:

1. Place a baking sheet or pizza stone into your oven and let your oven heat up to 500. DON'T take the baking sheet or pizza stone out of the oven while the oven heats.
2. Roll out your dough so that it creates a 13-inch circle, placing it on a piece of parchment so that it doesn't stick. Pierce the dough with a fork. Place the paper and dough onto the preheated stone—Bake for four minutes.
3. Pour the eight cups of water into a pot and allow it to come up to a boil. Place the asparagus and peas into the pot and cook for two minutes. Carefully remove, drain well, and immediately submerge them into some ice water so that they quit cooking. Allow them to drain and pat them with some paper towels to get rid of the excess water.
4. Mix together the garlic, coconut milk, and cashew ricotta. Mix this together well and spread it over the pizza dough. Leave a border of about one-half inch around the pizza.
5. Top with peas, asparagus, and vegan cheese. Let this cook for another ten minutes in the oven.
6. Put lemon juice and salt into a bowl. Place the zucchini "noodles" and toss them in the mixture so that they are well coated. Place on top of the pizza with the lemon zest, basil, and pepper. Cut into eight equal slices.

Day 9: Creamy mushroom risotto

Serves 4 | Prep 10min | Cook 35min | Total 45min

Ingredients:

- Pepper and salt
- Vegan butter 2 tbsp
- Vegetable stock, 6 c – divided (I prefer 3 tsp vegetable Better than Bouillon mixed in 3 c water)
- Arborio rice, 1.5 c – may use brown for max health but will change flavor
- Crushed garlic, 1 clove
- Cremini mushrooms, 5 c – for flavor I often sub 5 stalks chopped asparagus
- Chopped Vidalia onion
- Olive oil, 1 tbsp

Instructions:

1. Add the olive oil to a pot with the chopped onion and sauté on medium high for a couple of minutes until softened.
2. Add sliced mushrooms and garlic and toss with the onions.
3. Cover the pot and cook for a couple of minutes until the mushrooms have released some of their water.
4. Then remove the lid and add the rice and sauté it with the onions, mushrooms and garlic.
5. Then add 3 cups of vegetable stock, stir well, cover and simmer for around 20 minutes until the broth is mostly absorbed. *add asparagus with broth if not using mushrooms
6. Then add 1½ cups vegetable stock, stir well again, cover and simmer for around 10 minutes until the broth is mostly absorbed.
7. Then add a final 1 and ½ cups of vegetable stock, stir well again, cover and simmer for a final 5-10 minutes.
8. It's ready when all the stock has been mostly absorbed by the rice.

9. Turn off the heat and stir in the 2 Tbsp of vegan butter.
10. Add sea salt and black pepper to taste.
11. Serve it topped with fresh ground black pepper. Some vegan parmesan can also be really tasty sprinkled on top.

Day 10: Cuban Black Bean Soup

Serves 4 | Prep time: 30 min

Ingredients:

- o 4 cans (15 oz. each) Black Beans
- o 1 Tbsp. Olive Oil
- o 1 bottle (12 oz.) Beer
- o ½ cup Water
- o 1 Tbsp. Sherry, Dry
- o ¾ cup Onions, diced
- o ½ cup Green peppers, diced
- o 2 Tbsp. Garlic
- o ¼ tsp Ground Cumin
- o 2 tsp Tabasco sauce
- o To Taste Adobo seasoning, salt and pepper

Method:

1. Heat oil in a pot on medium heat.
2. Add the peppers, onions and garlic. Sauté for approximately 2 minutes.
3. Add the beer and Tabasco sauce, and bring to a boil.
4. Add 3 cans of beans with their juice and bring back to a boil.
5. Using a handheld kitchen blender, purée the soup until smooth.
6. Add the remaining 1 can of beans and bring back to a boil.

7. Add the Sherry wine, and season to taste with Adobo seasoning or salt and pepper.
8. Serve hot with steamed rice.

Variety is the spice of life so you could substitute dishes from Chapter 2 to go beyond ten days. If you are happy with your resultsthere are many vegan cookbooks out there and I plan to add a 30 day vegan cookbook to this book series.

Conclusion

Thank you for reading *The Whole Foods Plant Based Cookbook for Longevity* in *The Whole Foods Diet for Longevity Series*. The whole food plant-based diet is all about eating for a healthy, long, and strong life and can be started at any age to maximize your time with the ones you love. If you know anyone that's not well, eating this way has been shown to reverse many chronic diseases, reducing costly medications and side effects (see Chapter 2 in Book 1). In addition, whenever you cook any of these recipes, you are also eating for peak performance and helping the environment (see Chapters 4-5 in Book 1).

I hope you have found many savory recipes to add to your healthy meal prep, week in and week out. Perhaps they include Savory Sausage Pasta, Vegan Lasagna, Creamy Mushroom Risotto, Ultimate Chili, or Mom's Herb-Crusted Meatloaf. Mom's a former chef that says "Home cooking is cheaper, healthier, and tastier than eating out." Moreover, I hope this book has given you many options you need to reach your health goals, whatever those goals might be.

Remember you don't have to jump straight into this diet. You can make it easier on yourself by transitioning; some start out pescatarian and make slow changes until they reach a whole foods plant-based diet. Whatever you decide to do with your diet, it's important that you write it down and commit to it for at least ten straight days to see if it works for you. While there is a ten day meal plan here, you don't have to limit yourself to just ten days. You may find yourself enjoying higher energy levels and improved performance that will inspire you to lead a plant-based lifestyle long term.

"Be the change you want to see in the world." - *Gandhi*

Thank you

Thank you to you, the reader, for reading Book 2 in this series. If you find any of these tips or recipes helpful or just love a particular recipe, please share by leaving a review on Amazon:

https://www.amazon.com/review/create-review/?ie&asin=B0C87DH21W

It's through your support and reviews this book can help more people. Your review could help someone you know live healthy, long and strong. It may also help someone struggling to prepare fast, flavorful, filling recipes. Your valuable feedback will also help me with future editions and upcoming books in this series.

Thank you for reading!

Printed in Great Britain
by Amazon